Male Anorexia Nervosa

A Mother and Son's Journey

By Jon Sestak & Lynn Sestak

with Michelle Micsko, PhD.

Cover Photo by Bernadette Hursh @ brhursh.com

Contributions by Bailey Sestak and Steve Sestak

© 2016 Lynn and Jon Sestak

This book is a true story written from a personal perspective. This book is written as a source of information only and is not meant to be used to diagnose or treat eating disorders or other medical conditions. For diagnosis or treatment of eating disorders or other medical problems, please consult your own physician. The publisher and author are not responsible for any specific health needs that may require medical supervision and are not liable for any damages or negative consequences from any treatment, action, application or preparation, to any person reading or following the information in this book.

ACKNOWLEDGEMENT

We would like to thank Aline Zimmer who spent hours diligently editing this book for us. It was a lot of work dealing with these inexperienced writers. Thank you to our friends who supported us in this effort to inspire young men who suffer from anorexia nervosa to seek treatment and provide support and encouragement to those who love those men. Special thanks to Dr. Michelle Micsko for her expertise in the field and contribution to the book. Thank you to Leigh Cohn and Beth McGilley, PhD., who strive to create awareness of male eating disorders, for their encouragement. Tyler Moss, thank you for your advice. Finally, thank you to those who have supported Jon and our family during and after Jon's battle with anorexia nervosa. The phone calls and notes were appreciated.

CONTENTS

INTRODUCTION 1

PARENTAL INFLUENCE: LYNN 6

PARENTAL INFLUENCE: JON 11

YOUNGER YEAR INFLUENCE: LYNN 13

WARNING SIGNS: LYNN 18

EARLY TREATMENT: LYNN 25

INTENSIVE TREATMENT: LYNN 30

COMING TO TERMS: JON 39

PARTIAL INPATIENT TREATMENT: LYNN 45

PARTIAL INPATIENT TREATMENT: JON 50

TREATMENT: JON 54

ROAD TO RECOVERY: LYNN 57

ROAD TO RECOVERY: JON 60

RELATIONSHIPS: JON 64

LIFE TODAY: LYNN 68

LIFE TODAY: JON 71

DR. MICHELLE MICSKO'S PERSPECTIVE 76

BAILEY'S PERSPECTIVE 91

STEVE'S PERSPECTIVE 94

SUPPORTIVE BIBLE VERSES   99

REFERENCES   102

BIOGRAPHY   105

INTRODUCTION

Have you been touched by an eating disorder affecting a male family member or friend? Are you feeling hurt or closed off in your relationship, hopeless, angry, frustrated, desperate, powerless, or sad? Chances are you are predominantly worried and searching for ways you can help and support him. We commend you for your effort in finding out more about the disease. Whether it is reading recommended books, learning from reputable websites, or speaking to a dietician, physician, or therapist trained in treating clients with anorexia nervosa, we hope you find the tools you need to support and seek treatment for those you love and care about.

From Jon:

Before I was diagnosed as a sufferer of anorexia nervosa, I was an outsider to addiction. I looked at addiction as a disease that was self-evoked, a habit or act carried out in a manner which becomes detrimental to one's health either emotionally or physically. I felt this throughout my eating disorder, often blaming myself for having inflicted the disease on myself. After the eating disorder took over my body, it was as if the former me no longer existed. As my weight dropped, I drowned deeper and deeper behind the darkness of the eating disorder. I kept losing friends due to the isolation my disease insisted on, and I felt no pain. If you have never gone through an addiction, you cannot understand the type and amount of control it has over your mind and body, which is why it is so hard to overcome. It is not because you are naïve, but because it is something you must experience to understand. This was the case for my friends, families, and others who wanted so desperately to help me. They couldn't possibly fathom the control and power the eating disorder had over their son, friend, nephew, brother, or grandchild.

From Lynn:

If you are a mother of a son with anorexia nervosa, know you are not alone. Personally, I have never felt as helpless, lonely, and afraid as when my son, Jon, suffered from restrictive type anorexia nervosa. The disease was killing him, shutting down his organs, and taking over his mind. Jon was enduring the detrimental physical and psychological effects of the disease and painfully aware of the emotional hurt the disease inflicted upon those who loved him. Feeling blamed and responsible, I grew emotionally distant from family and friends and focused on trying to help and protect my son from unwarranted judgment while getting him the medical treatment he required. Those closest to us had difficulty understanding and frankly, the reasons for the behaviors associated with the disease are difficult to explain to others and challenging to comprehend unless you have experienced it. Even in group therapy sessions with other parents and sufferers, we felt alone because Jon was the only male in his groups during the majority of his treatment. There was only one other young man Jon met in treatment during the course of his nearly three-year intensive battle, making some aspects of our experience with a male affliction difficult to share with others and vice versa.

By the grace of God, Jon did survive. He maintains a healthy weight and exercise routine and bravely shares his story with others. We have an open, honest, and closer relationship as a family, and he has restored broken friendships and made new ones along the way. Best of all, we all have a renewed faith in the power of God. This book's intent is to provide you with hope, support, strengthened faith, and resources as we share our journey and sometimes brutally honest experiences from a mother and son's perspective.

Anorexia nervosa IS a disease. It is not a choice. It is not rebellion. It is not a result of poor parenting. It is not a self-centered child looking for attention.

According to The National Association for Males with Eating Disorders ("Anorexia Nervosa", 2016), anorexia nervosa is most centrally characterized by an intense fear of gaining weight (or becoming fat) with a consequent failure to maintain an adequate body weight due to dietary restricting. It may also include body image disturbance. Additionally, anorexia nervosa may feature periodic binge eating and/or purging (e.g., self-induced vomiting, laxative or diuretic use), or compulsive exercise. Whilst males are generally less affected than women, emerging research shows that anorexia nervosa in males is increasing. However, it is important to note that alongside reporting a drive for thinness and a desire to be thin, males with anorexia nervosa may also report a desire to be 'lean' or 'ripped', with similar symptomatic features.

According to a review of numerous studies by Mond, Mitchison, & Hay (2014), for activities such as binge eating, 42-45% of bingers were male; as were 28-100% of individuals who regularly purged. Laxative abuse among genders was nearly even, and fasting for weight loss was endorsed by nearly 40% of the males.

Anorexia has the highest mortality rate of all mental disorders, with a mortality rate of 5% per decade. Young people ages 15-24 years with anorexia have 10 times the risk of dying compared to their same age (Fichter & Quadflieg, 2016; Smink, & Hoek, 2012). The National Eating Disorder Association reports up to 20% mortality rate among individuals who suffer from anorexia nervosa. According to a study by Steinhausen (2002), of 5590 patients diagnosed with anorexia nervosa, among those who survived, on average less than one-half recovered, one-third improved, and 20% remained chronically ill. Another study found over an 8% mortality rate among male patients (Gueguen et al., 2012). Sources agree that the sooner it is diagnosed and treatment begun, the better the chances of success. However, prevalence of eating disorders in males is greater than estimated because men are often too stigmatized to seek treatment for "women's problems" (Cohn, 2013).

The following are statistics involving males with eating disorders according to the National Eating Disorders Association:

- The most widely-quoted study estimates that males have a lifetime prevalence of .3% for anorexia nervosa (AN), .5% for bulimia nervosa (BN) and 2% for binge eating disorder (BED). These figures correspond to males representing 25% of individuals with AN and BN and 36% of those with BED. They are based on DSM-IV criteria (Hudson, Hiripi, Pope, & Kessler, 2007)

- In the United States, 20 million women and 10 million men will suffer from a clinically significant eating disorder at some time in their life, including anorexia nervosa, bulimia nervosa, binge eating disorder, or EDNOS [EDNOS is now recognized as OSFED, other specified feeding or eating disorder, per the DSM-5] (Wade, Keski-Rahkonen, & Hudson, 2011)

- In a study of 1,383 adolescents, the prevalence of any DSM-5 ED in males was reported to be 1.2% at 14 years, 2.6% at 17 years, and 2.9% at 20 years (Allen, Byrne, Oddy, & Crosby, 2013)

- A study of 2,822 students on a large university campus found that 3.6% of males had positive screens for ED. The female-to-male ratio was 3-to-1 (Eisenberg, Nicklett, Roeder, & Kirz, 2011)

- In looking at male sexuality and eating disorders, a higher percentage of gay (15%) than heterosexual males (5%) had diagnoses of ED, but when these percentages are applied to population figures, the majority of males with ED are heterosexual (Feldman & Meyer, 2007)

- Various studies suggest that risk of mortality for males with ED is higher than it is for females (Raevuoni, Keski-Rahkonen, & Hoek, 2014)

- Men with eating disorders often suffer from comorbid conditions such as depression, excessive exercise, substance disorders, and anxiety (Weltzin et al., 2014b)

PARENTAL INFLUENCE: Lynn

We consider ourselves a typical, Christian, Midwestern family with strong family roots. We raised two kids and a dog, none of whom are perfect, including the parents. My husband, Steve, and I have been married for over 25 years. We have a son and a daughter. Jon's sister, Bailey, is 16 months his younger. At the time of Jon's illness, we had a beloved dog named Bagel. She was a Blenheim Cavalier King Charles Spaniel. The only name the kids at ages 7 and 8 could agree on was Bagel surmising that she looked like a toasted bagel with cream cheese, a common breakfast item at our house at the time. I find this ironic that we now avoid formerly favorite foods because the carbohydrate has been demonized and considered "bad".

My husband, Steve, is a successful business owner who traveled during much of our children's early years. Although raised to be calm and stoic in times of stress or sadness, he wasn't a distant dad. When he was home, he went to activities, coached Jon in soccer, roughhoused, and loved on the kids with frequent hugs, positive reinforcement, and the beloved belly bomb when it was time for bed. I, too, am a hugger and nurturing mother unafraid to show emotion or share an opinion, solicited or unsolicited. Early in my career I was a physical therapist with a private practice which allowed me flexibility with the kids. However, when the kids were ages two and three, we chose to follow Steve's promising career path and move away from extended family. We made the decision for me to stay at home to raise the kids, manage the household, and work PRN at a hospital. I stopped practicing physical therapy when they were late into elementary school and later began what I consider "*hobby*" businesses, none of which place me on the front of Time but which I enjoy nonetheless.

When I chose to stay home, I took the job of parenting very seriously, structuring days similar to the preschools when the kids were young and jumping into the PTA, booster clubs, and community organizations when the kids began school. Those days provided the opportunities to interact not only with our kids but with their friends, teachers, coaches, and teammates. Whether it was chatting during carpools, organizing events with friends, tutoring students, volunteering, or watching the numerous sporting events, I enjoyed the variety.

Although I loved being a part of their lives and felt blessed for the opportunity to stay at home, I often struggled with the social stigma when out with adults. I tried to shrug off insensitive stay-at-home mom comments and my hurt feelings when conversations centered on unreciprocated questions about my work and life interests that challenged my self-esteem. I often didn't feel valued and resented my husband's travel that prevented me from a full time career and the corresponding paycheck, social status, and independence. I would leave engagements discouraged by feigned interest in my volunteer efforts in the community or a conversation to stretch my intellectual bones. I felt others only saw me as my husband's wife who did nothing but stay at home and probably spend "his" money.

There were many awkward moments when meeting someone and the inevitable question was asked, "What type of work do you do?" and then appear stuck for a follow up question when I answered, "I manage the household and raise the kids." There was always that hope of a validating follow up question such as, "Oh, do you volunteer on any committees at school or community organizations?" hoping for a connection outside of careers. I began adding, "In my previous life I was a physical therapist but now I stay home and raise the kids," which often sparked questions about my one-time paying job but further validated the stereotype of the career that I loved most. I often envied those with careers that allowed them to travel or work outside the home because sometimes my only adult conversation for the day would be the casual greeting from clerks during those titillating trips to the grocery store. As the saying goes, the grass is always greener on the other side.

The patented "I would love to help with (insert activity), but I work" comment when asking others to volunteer for their child's event would feed the low self-esteem. I felt sad and angry at the same time for their kids. "Really?" I would think. Work is so important that you can't engage your kids in frosting store-bought sugar cookies for half an hour, pick up some paper plates at the store, or volunteer at a dance? Yep. Those were my judgement days, stemming from pure pride and insecurity.

I am sharing this not because I thought I was a perfect mom playing martyr or passing judgement on working parents. Far from it! The painful truth is I didn't value myself. The kids and their activities and achievements were idols in my life. I chose to feed my insecurities by minimizing my value and carrying that chip on my shoulder. When asked, "What do you do?" I shouldn't have stopped at, "I manage the household and raise the kids." I could have said something more along the lines, "With my husband traveling as much as he does, we feel that it is important for one of us to hold down the fort and make sure the house doesn't burn to the ground so I have become involved in (insert organization) and currently I am working on (insert project)."

Some women identify with their career, salaries, and social status which may be their idols. My identity and idols became the children and volunteer activities, and my insecurities flourished. The sin of insecurity thrived as a young mom concerned more about what others thought of me and my parenting than of how God wanted me to serve for His glorification. I wondered if I would feel more accepted if I worked full time, worried about passing down my insecurities to the kids, and feared stunting their independence by being too involved in their daily lives.

You never know others' circumstances and shouldn't judge them for not managing life like you. We should support one another, especially as women. I am not proud of those thoughts and have grown a lot in my relationship with Christ since those days. Although there are still struggles, my security no longer rests in what I do or what others think of me, and I try not to judge others for not being excited about things that I have a passion or responding in a way I had hoped.

I preface our story with my insecurity trait because one of the recurring arguments Jon and I had when he was in high school revolved around my bringing ice cream, cookies, or some other snack du jour down to the basement where the kids hung out when they had friends over. I loved watching the kids dive into the treats like they had never seen a cookie before and thought Jon's feelings of annoyance were misplaced. It wasn't the food that bothered him, but rather the interaction with his friends. I never understood at the time why he lashed out at me. After all, it wasn't like I plopped down next to his friends on the couch and spent the evening with them. What could possibly be the problem?

He also wasn't thrilled when I chaired the school dances one year in high school and had to be present at two of them. I never saw him in the throng of dancers, of course; but, in his mind he knew I was there lurking behind the refreshment table, certain to ruin his evening. What I saw as my purpose to serve others and be the Kool Aid mom, Jon clearly saw as a lack of trust and an infringement on his right to privacy. And the truth of the matter is I did trust him. He had never given me reason not to trust him. It hit me hard when he yelled at me once as he was storming out of the house, "Mom, you say it's for me but it's never for me. It's for you!" Ouch! There was certainly some truth to that statement.

Don't get me wrong. I wasn't the overprotective, indulging mom like the one on the Goldbergs sitcom but I can relate to the mom on Modern Family. Not the confident, bombshell character, unfortunately, but the other one with her control and struggles with insecurity characteristics.

I don't regret being involved. I just wish I was more confident in my role. I really found joy during my time volunteering and serving where there were needs. There are some really great memories working with friends and getting to know the teachers, coaches, and kids. And my involvement didn't seem to bother my daughter. We didn't have arguments like those I had with Jon. However, I will always wonder if I wasn't listening to my son's needs clearly enough as his independence matured, and if my selfish desire to feel worthy factored into his suffering from anorexia nervosa.

PARENTAL INFLUENCE: Jon

Humans are doers. They are problem-solvers. When a problem arises, it is their inclination to try and solve the problem by any means necessary. A prime example would be my father. My father has always been my role model. He is hard working, humble, and always seemed to succeed. It is very typical for a boy to look up to his father. Today I can still say that during my life there has never been a single moment when I questioned who my biggest role model is. I have always admired my father for who he is as a person and not for what he has accomplished, but how he has accomplished it.

When I was stricken with this disorder, it was my dad's intuition that there must be a fix. He tried everything in his power to make the eating disorder subside. During the time the eating disorder was at its peak, I often saw my father's fear and worry translate into anger. "Why could he not help his son?" The answer is so easy "just eat," but deep down I knew that although the answer seemed simple, the illness would not be resolved so easily. He did not express his anger, but bottled it internally. Our time together was often interrupted by the eating disorder which severely affected our relationship. I don't know exactly how to explain our relationship during this time except to say that I wasn't always present. Days together were usually "speed bumped" by meal times and food selections.

My mother is also a doer, but the core of her approach is in the understanding of a problem. She analyzes it and then seeks a solution that is logical and reasonable. I think it comes primarily from her background. My mother was always a hard-working, dedicated student who went the extra mile to achieve the highest grade. She was the "involved" mom, always volunteering for school and classroom activities. At the time, I dreaded seeing my mom at school for fear of embarrassment. It wasn't until I attended college that I fully appreciated the role my mom played in my life outside of home. So when it came to my illness, she sought every available resource and outlet to try and understand what her son was dealing with.

The difficulty with eating disorders is that men and women get the disease from a variety of factors, and the best method of treatment varies from person to person. For me, it took a life-altering experience to open a tiny outlet for Jon to look at himself and see what he had become. I met another recovered girl, at a treatment center I visited, where recovery was spurred by a bribe from her parents. Everyone is different.

My mom often was frustrated by the reality that there is not just one right answer. During my struggle, my parents consulted a therapist in hope of trying to understand the disease. My mom read books and online resources to gain information. In the end, she realized that there is no one protocol to cure anorexia. It comes in all shapes and sizes; therefore, you need to alter your approach accordingly. Although it pained her to come to this conclusion, she realized that the only thing she could do was offer further support while she watched her son suffer and, involuntarily, almost take his own life.

YOUNGER YEAR INFLUENCE: Lynn

Jon was a typical boy growing up. He was a good student, carrying A's and B's. He exceled at math, preferring the challenges it presented over learning a foreign language any day. Grades were never an argument, although his father and I were always amazed at his ability to determine precisely, to the tenth of a percent, what he required on his final exam to get that A or B grade. If an A seemed too hard to reach with, say, a 94 percent requirement, he seemed happy to settle for the B. A common personality characteristic of students who suffer from anorexia nervosa is striving for perfection in school. This wasn't true with our son. However, it was Jon's striving for perfection on the athletic field where we spotted the first warning signs.

Always one of the smaller kids in school, Jon felt an intense need to prove himself on the field. Growing up, he was in the 50th percentile in weight and the 25th in height. As described by one of his elementary teachers, he was one of the "sporty" boys who played at recess. He loved sports and STILL loves sports. He was one of two of the shorter "sporty" boys in his friend group. On a side note, the boys in his class seemed to be particularly gifted with size and height, a bunch of young Herculean characters! Two of his friends ended up receiving scholarships and doing quite well in college sports, one in swimming and the other, Drew, as a tight end in football at the University of Minnesota. Looking back at pictures, we notice how, intended or not, Jon always ended up next to the tallest kid. Elementary school picture days were always a disappointment for Jon as he was inevitably placed in the dreaded front row.

He endured teasing about being small. I remember one friend affectionately calling him "alien head" because he thought his body was disproportionate to his head. As a coping mechanism, Jon developed a wonderful sense of humor at a young age. Fortunately, classmates also recognized his athletic ability and outgoing nature. He was a pretty good basketball shot and had some wheels on him.

This, combined with his witty sense of humor and intelligence, kept the bullying to a minimum. All in all, he made some really good friends who all matured into fine young men.

Jon's speed became the attribute that helped him the most athletically. After exposure to numerous sports, musical instruments, and various activities over the years, soccer became the activity that stuck. He played confidently in the defensive back position where his speed, strength, and smaller stature stood him well on the soccer field where he played year round.

His only major emotional setback pertaining to soccer was a rejection by the coach of the team on which two close friends played in elementary school. He had tried out for their team and was told he was skilled enough but too small. Unfortunately, that was also the same time his best buddy from the neighborhood, Jaret, moved across the country, followed shortly after by another friend. That was a really tough year for him. He struggled socially because all of his friends lived outside the neighborhood. If he wanted to hang out with them, we had to drive him. These boys also played on basketball and baseball teams together, so it wasn't second nature for them to include Jon, especially during the summer. It was a time before cellphones were the norm. The days of stepping outside to join friends shooting hoops or kicking the ball around in the commons area had come to an end. My heart ached for my son so many times during that year.

With the help of his fifth and sixth grade teachers, Mrs. Wilcoxson and Mrs. Waters, he began to bounce back and gain more confidence. Contact lenses replaced his glasses. Friendships strengthened. He transferred to another premier soccer team which he enjoyed, meshing with the defensive guys and appreciating the hard work and personalities of the coaches. We liked the team as well. The coaches were supportive, provided good instruction, and the team did well competitively. We also moved that year to a new neighborhood closer to his friends and other children his age.

Looking back, I again wonder what childhood factors, if any, contributed to the groundwork for his anorexia. Researchers have concluded there are a variety of reasons why eating disorders strike. They identify common psychological factors such as control and coping skills, social and family issues, genetic, and environmental factors that create a "perfect storm" for it to strike. Every case is unique.

When I reflect on Jon's early and teen years, I would say some factors that played a part include low self-esteem due to his small stature which he disguised with humor, a history of being teased, a lack of control due to my involvement and others' perceptions of him, anxiety related to performance, and mild depression (undiagnosed), anger, stress, and loneliness stemming from the year when he didn't make the soccer team and his friends moved away. There are also familial genetic components of anxiety disorders such as claustrophobia, perfectionism, and depression. I see now that the breakup with his first high school love, combined with the stress of heading off to college and his inability to express his emotions, may have been factors as well. During his illness, I asked Jon if he had been sexually abused. He assured me that he had not. Although he exhibited several of the eating disorder factors outlined below, he only exhibited the low BMI of the isolated factors identified specifically for anorexia nervosa. He was born at a healthy weight; however, he fell off the growth chart for a short period of time as a young toddler, when he suffered from rectal prolapses.

Below are factors outlined by the National Eating Disorders Association (Jones, n.d.) that can contribute to eating disorders:

Biological

- Possible imbalance of chemicals in the brain that control hunger, appetite, and digestion
- Current research indicates there are significant genetic contributions

Psychological

- Low self-esteem
- Feelings of inadequacy or lack of control in life
- Depression, anxiety, anger, stress, or loneliness

Interpersonal

- Troubled personal relationships
- Difficulty expressing emotions and feelings
- History of being teased or ridiculed based on size or weight
- History of physical or sexual abuse

Social

- Cultural pressures that glorify "thinness" or muscularity and place value on obtaining the "perfect body"
- Narrow definitions of beauty that include only women and men of specific body weights and shapes
- Cultural norms that value people on the basis of physical appearance and not inner qualities and strengths
- Stress related to racial, ethnic, size/weight-related or other forms of discrimination or prejudice

A specific factor identified for anorexia nervosa is a low body mass index (BMI) and some smaller studies indicate the following risk factors associated to anorexia nervosa:

- Childhood eating conflicts
- Struggles around meals
- Vaginal instrumental delivery
- Cephalohematoma – collection of blood beneath the periosteum of the newborn's skull
- Premature birth
- Low birth weight

- Delivery of multiple babies at once
- Perfectionism

WARNING SIGNS: Lynn

During his high school years, Jon was well liked and hardworking. He was a good student, a member of the National Honor Society, and participated in numerous clubs. He was truly and unexpectedly honored by his 400-plus classmates as a Homecoming candidate and joked to me while I proudly stood next to him on the court as they announced the second runner-up, "I'm out!" Two of his "sporty" elementary school friends, Drew and A.J., were named first runner-up and king. He was sincerely happy for them and so was I. It was a lovely memory for mother and son. And his first love mentioned earlier, whom we adored as well, became the Homecoming queen. Jon will still say that Homecoming and the surrounding events were among his favorite memories of high school.

He played soccer all his life, making the junior varsity squad as a freshman and honored to be a team captain of the varsity soccer team his senior year along with two of his childhood best friends, Adam and Kyle. His premier and high school teams made State playoff runs both years on varsity, and Jon was referred to by a television sports commentator during a playoff game as a "bulldog," which he embraced. He also ran track all four years of high school, with his team winning State his senior year.

He had a close group of friends who made good decisions the majority of the time. In fact, we vacationed with several of their families for spring breaks. We enjoyed the parents and siblings as well. Coincidentally, Jon's closest friends in high school also had siblings our daughter's age who were very close and remain so to this day.

Always seeking work opportunities, Jon held several jobs and created some entrepreneurial opportunities beginning at age 14. He worked in the food industry and wasn't afraid of manual labor: pulling weeds, spreading mulch, and other miscellaneous jobs that most kids would shy away. For him and his friend, Adam, it was hard work but great money.

He had been accepted to his school of choice, Saint Louis University (SLU). Everything had gone so well for him these past several years. So what happened?

The disease starts so innocently. Males often work to improve their body image through weight lifting and body building as they try to become stronger and more athletic.

ANAD identifies the following statistics pertaining to athletes:

- Risk Factors: In judged sports – sports that score participants – prevalence of eating disorders is 13% (compared with 3% in refereed sports) (Zucker, Womble, Williamson, & Perrin, 1999)

- Significantly higher rates of eating disorders found in elite athletes (20%) than in a female control group (9%) (Sungot-Borgen, &Torstveit, 2004)

- Female athletes in aesthetic sports (e.g. gymnastics, ballet, figure skating) found to be at the highest risk for eating disorders (Sungot-Borgen, & Torstveit, 2004)

- A comparison of the psychological profiles of athletes and those with anorexia found these factors in common: perfectionism, high self-expectations, competitiveness, hyperactivity, repetitive exercise routines, compulsiveness, drive, tendency toward depression, body image distortion, preoccupation with dieting and weight (Bachner-Melman, Zohar, Ebstein, Elizur, & Constantini, 2006)

Eating disorder beginnings are often described as a switch being flipped. What starts out as an effort to improve weight or fitness goes awry. This is how it was with my son. He began struggling his senior year during spring track season. Underclassmen who were faster than he was replaced him on the 4 x 100 and eventually the 4 x 400. Jon, in an effort to improve, began doing extra workouts at home, running hills, sprinting, and practicing starts. He also began focusing more on what he was eating and set a goal of participating in a long-course triathlon. At the same time, he and his girlfriend were working through their relationship as they headed off to different colleges in the fall and were unwittingly dealing with some psychological changes that had begun from the disease already. Little did we know the switch had been flipped.

According to Weltzin (2014a), over 50% of males presenting for eating disorder treatment at Rogers Memorial Hospital report problematic exercise behaviors. He referred to a study by Hausenblas & Downs (2002) that, compared to women, men are more susceptible to elements of excessive exercise such as a lack of control, increased tolerance, and reduction in alternative activities. According to Weltzin, signs of excessive exercise include highly structured and repetitive exercise routines that tend to focus more on endurance activities, most commonly running. Patients will often engage in exercise rather than spend time with family or attend school or work. Furthermore, continuing to engage in exercise even when injured or while underweight is common. Increased emotional distress when exercise is limited is common. Also, excessive exercising tends to occur alone or in secret.

Why am I focusing so much on sports? Were we the parents who berated the coaches, refs, and our own child after a loss? Did we insist on Jon trying out and participating for only winning teams? If you asked anyone, including Jon, I hope they would say that we weren't perfect but didn't have a reputation of being *"those"* parents. Did we want Jon to be on teams where the players were kids who were nice and didn't play dirty, with coaches who didn't yell, and teams that won more than they lost? Of course. Car rides were a lot more fun heading home after a win.

I might add the same went for the classroom. We wanted Jon to be in a classroom where he was challenged but not overwhelmed, with a teacher who enjoyed teaching and was able to adapt to his learning style, and with classmates who, too, wanted to learn. We didn't expect A's but knew he was capable of A's and B's which were never a problem for him.

However, I might emphasize a point of wisdom I've gained from reflection. I think we, as parents, can inadvertently create in a child an attitude of inadequacy, or fear of disappointment. In an effort to help our child succeed, we may unwittingly put pressure on them by seeking out the "best" teams or the "best" schools or the "best" sorority or fraternity in college. Sometimes we need to let kids fail and not save them from an occasional disappointment. It's part of life. It's part of learning. It's part of maturation. We should guide them but not do the work for them. Let them take ownership and actively establish their own future and goals and be involved in activities because THEY want to be a part, not because of our dreams for them or because it looks good on a resume. We need to encourage them to engage in their passion and their purpose. How much do academic and athletic wins and losses at those young ages really matter in the big picture of life? How the kids respond to those challenges, successes, and failures, how coaches respond, and how you respond will shape your child.

Parents, coaches, teachers, friends, coworkers, relatives, and even professional sportsmen, actors, and government officials, all help shape the lives of those around us by our behavior. Make it count for the better. Most kids are hard enough on themselves. They want to be a part of something they can connect with. Most of all, they want to feel love and respect. We need to build them up, not tear them down, so they CAN be part of the greater good and fulfill what God has planned for them.

In fact, I remember a poignant moment between Jon and me when we were walking to the car after a soccer loss. He was young and playing for his first team. The team was not doing well, losing quite a few games after moving up a division. I tried to console Jon and tell him what I thought a parent would say in a situation like this. "It's okay. Winning isn't everything, Jon. You did your best." I will never forget him turning to me and saying, "Yeah, but it's nice to win sometimes, mom." I couldn't argue. Jon was and is a very driven young man. Most kids with eating disorders are. He wants to succeed and doesn't want to let anyone down, especially his teammates, friends, coworkers, and family. Like I said, most kids are harder on themselves. Okay. I will climb down off of my high horse now.

The signs of anorexia nervosa began around the beginning of April of his senior year of high school but I wasn't putting them together at the time. He was asking me a lot about foods and recipes. He took an interest in healthy options and began keeping a recipe book on his own. I also noted that he started cutting down first on fats and then on carbohydrates in his diet. Exercise grew excessive over the next couple of months. By summer, he had signed up to participate in his first triathlon. He would run, swim, and bike all in one day and seemed to be restless if he wasn't doing something. My husband and I noticed fairly early that he was losing some weight. Jon acknowledged he had lost a few pounds but said it was unintentional which we believed to be true. We thought he just needed to eat more food to balance his exercise routine. Concerned he was training too hard for the triathlon, we encouraged him to contact a close friend, Cathy Wood, who is an elite, well-respected triathlete regarding his training. That was a nice effort but, in hindsight, we should have been consulting healthcare professionals. We thought a little guidance would help get him on track with his training. We just didn't know what was going on at this point.

We also noticed his emotions would fluctuate. He began feeling disappointment deeper. For instance, he would apologize after a track race when he didn't place. Knowing how hard he was trying, we felt bad for him but we never were upset or disappointed in his track performances, and neither were his coaches, from what we could tell. The track team was full of camaraderie and support. We loved watching the kids run from one side of the track to the other, cheering on their teammates during long races. When Jon was racing, it was no different. And even though his times had increased and he had lost his positions in the relays his senior year as he got weaker, Coach Cooper still recognized him as a leader, asked him to assist him, and took him to State as an alternate, where they brought home the title. Jon said he didn't feel like a contributor to the team by that point, however.

In late April or May, he came to me complaining about a painful hip. I laid him down and used my physical therapy skills to evaluate him. When I saw that his gluteal muscles had atrophied, I became concerned. As a soccer player and sprinter, he always had a muscular gluteal region. He had always been very fit with a low fat percentage and a good muscular build. Now, his muscles had completely wasted away around his hip. It was at this point that I connected the dots – restrictive eating, low self-esteem, mood swings, excessive exercise, preoccupation with food, and weight loss were the primary symptoms. By early summer, he had developed all the warning signs outlined by the National Eating Disorders Association (NEDA) and National Association of Anorexia Nervosa and Associated Disorders (ANAD) for male anorexia nervosa. However, not suspecting anorexia until now, I had never been on the websites.

In May, I took him to his pediatrician where the diagnosis was confirmed by history, blood tests, EKG, and physical exam. The main concern at this point was bradycardia which is an abnormally slow heart rate. At this early stage in the disease, Jon recognized that there was a problem but was in denial. He acknowledged all of these things but really didn't feel like it was something to worry about, nor did his dad. In fact, because we had an early diagnosis, we thought it would be cured quickly before he left for college. We had no idea what this disease was about to do to our son.

The National Eating Disorders Association provides the following warning signs for anorexia nervosa ("Anorexia Nervosa Warning Signs," n.d.)

- Dramatic weight loss

- Preoccupation with weight, food, calories, fat grams, and dieting

- Refusal to eat certain foods, progressing to restrictions against whole categories of food (e.g. no carbohydrates, etc.)

- Frequent comments about feeling "fat" or overweight despite weight loss

- Anxiety about gaining weight or being "fat"

- Denial of hunger

- Development of food rituals (e.g. eating foods in certain orders, excessive chewing, rearranging food on a plate)

- Consistent excuses to avoid mealtimes or situations involving food

- Excessive, rigid exercise regimen--despite weather, fatigue, illness, or injury, the need to "burn off" calories taken in

- Withdrawal from usual friends and activities

- In general, behaviors and attitudes indicating that weight loss, dieting, and control of food are becoming primary concerns

EARLY TREATMENT: Lynn

The National Eating Disorders Association lists five Stages of Change in the recovery process defined by Prochaska and DiClemente: Pre-contemplation, Contemplation, Preparation, Action, and Maintenance (Brotsky, 2014).

- The Pre-contemplation Stage is evident when a person does not believe she has a problem. Those who are close to him pick up on symptoms such as restrictive eating, the binge/purge cycle, or a preoccupation with weight, shape, and appearance even before the individual admits to it. He may refuse to discuss the topic and deny he needs help. At this stage, it is necessary to gently educate the individual about the devastating effects the disorder will have on his health and life, and the positive aspects of change.

- The Contemplation Stage occurs when the individual is willing to admit that she has a problem and is now open to receiving help. The fear of change may be very strong, and it is during this phase that a psychotherapist should assist the individual in discovering the function of her eating disorder so she can understand why it is in her life and how it no longer serves her. This, in turn, helps the individual in moving closer toward the next stage of change.

- The person transitions into the Preparation Stage when she is ready to change, but is uncertain about how to do it. Time is spent establishing specific coping skills such as appropriate boundary setting and assertiveness, effective ways of dealing with negative eating disorder thoughts and emotions, and ways to tend to her personal needs. Potential barriers to change are identified. A plan of action is developed by the treatment team, (i.e. psychotherapist, nutritionist, and physician) as well as the individual and designated family members. Generally, a list of people to call during times of crisis is created at this juncture.

- The Action Stage begins when the person is ready to implement her strategy and confront the eating disorder behavior head on. At this point, she is open to trying new ideas and behaviors and willing to face fears in order for the change to occur. Trusting the treatment team and her support network is essential to making the Action Stage successful.

- The Maintenance Stage evolves when the person has sustained the Action Stage for approximately six months or longer. During this period, she is actively practicing her new behaviors and new ways of thinking as well as consistently using both healthy self-care and coping skills. Part of this stage also includes revisiting potential triggers in order to prevent relapse, establishing new areas of interests, and beginning to live her life in a meaningful way.

After receiving the diagnosis of anorexia nervosa from his doctor, we were referred to the Renew Counseling Center which is a local program for eating disorders. At that time, it was the only program available in Kansas City. Unfortunately, as with all clinics we encountered, there was a waiting list to begin treatment. The first visit wasn't until August 2nd. Before Jon left for college, he was only able to schedule and attend three dietician and four therapist appointments. In this early stage, the therapists didn't recommend that we keep him home from college but did recommend continued treatment while he was at college.

During the same period, one family counseling session was scheduled so learning about the disease was very new and overwhelming to my husband and me. This is where we were stunned to learn about the eating disorder (ED) and specifically the anorexia nervosa that was taking over our son's body and mind. It was about this same time my husband came around to realize this was a serious problem and not simply a matter of Jon losing weight solely from training and just having mood swings. Jon was addicted to exercise. Steve had spent his career problem solving. The solution was simple to him. You lose too much weight; you take in more calories. I don't want to brush over this point. One of the things that was vitally important to help Jon was for Steve and me to be on the same page. Just like a child will do when he wants to go out with friends or wants you to buy him something, ED will seek out the weak one in a situation and exploit your emotions and feelings of guilt without hesitation.

I would encourage you to share the NEDA, ANAD, and NAMED (National Association for Males with Eating Disorders) websites with those closest to you who will encounter your son and even encourage them to schedule a counseling session with a trained professional. The more effort loved ones take to understand the disease, the more effective support they can provide and possibly avoid their feelings being hurt during the course of the disease. The disease will affect every aspect of the sufferer's life, including close relationships.

As the disease progressed, withdrawal was probably the most commonly noted component by friends and family. Jon rarely went out with friends and avoided family gatherings. And if a meal was involved? You would think we were taking him to a torture chamber with the anxiety that ensued. The professionals advised us to encourage him and not force him to eat or participate in activities. These had to be his choices. The sad thing is, Jon knew how much the behaviors were affecting those who loved him, and it upset him. He never wanted to disappoint anybody. But ED had its grip on him and was holding tight.

Emotionally, we couldn't help but limit our time away from him because of our concern for his health as we saw the disease taking its toll. I was scared to leave the house after his first year of college. I know that sounds dramatic, but the fear of him suffering a heart attack during a swim in the lake or during a secret run at night was very real for me. Our son's health was our priority. If we weren't around him, we felt he wasn't going to make an effort to eat and would definitely exercise excessively. The behaviors and our need to protect Jon often provoked anger and hurt feelings by those around us who had difficulty understanding.

When we tried to explain the disease manifestations and Jon's need for support, not criticism, we received responses such as "He eats fine when he is with us," "We don't have any anxiety on our side of the family," "It's just a phase," or my personal favorite, "Maybe it is because you favor Bailey more." People may want to try to pinpoint a reason for his illness and lash out when they are hurt by the behavior. You should expect it and not be surprised. It is important to forgive and not feel blame. Trust me. You will beat yourself up enough. Remember, the disease and all of its intricacies of treatment and irrational behaviors are hard enough for us closest to it to understand. Don't expect others to understand it any better. These are important times to give it to God and pray.

Jon went ahead and raced in the triathlon he had been training for since spring of his senior year. The race took place prior to beginning treatment and learning more about the disease. Our pleas to pull out fell on deaf ears. We went to watch and support him. I remember feeling very torn as a mom. Was I supporting him or going to watch him die that day? I remember Jon refusing to pray with me for his safety before getting out of the car. It didn't stop me. I spent a lot of time in prayer that day. The entire time, I feared he would pass out or suffer a heart attack and the ambulance would rush him off to the hospital. Thankfully, he was able to finish and ate a huge breakfast afterward with us. My husband and I thought maybe now that the triathlon is over, THIS will be his turning point. HA!

Subsequently that summer, I got my hands on every resource I could find so I could try to understand more about the disease. A friend whose daughter survived anorexia was able to recommend several books and the information on the NEDA and ANAD websites was quite helpful. Most information and studies, however, pertain to females. Specific information was scarce regarding male anorexia. Although 10 million men are estimated to suffer from anorexia, most resources point out that males are less likely to be diagnosed early or at all, may feel shame regarding the diagnosis so don't seek treatment, and have a tendency to delay treatment.

We quickly realized that the treatment was a marathon, not a sprint, and things would get much worse before they got better, if they did at all. We learned that ED would continue to wedge into his mind and control his emotions, thoughts, and behavior. Worst of all, we knew this eating disorder could take his life. We began to really despise ED and realized how important it was to differentiate ED from Jon. ED was evil. Jon was our beloved son who we would do anything for to save his life. Jon told me he didn't like me to refer to ED but there were times when the overwhelming frustration was so strong that it was the only way I could cope and keep liking my son. Please note what I just said. I always loved Jon but not the effect ED had on him. Separating the two was important for me and a useful coping tool.

INTENSIVE TREATMENT: Lynn

As with most parents, we felt a double edged sword as we took him to college. He was excited to go off to Saint Louis University (SLU). He was our first child in college and we experienced the pangs of dropping him off. Whether they were at a natural or unnatural level, I couldn't tell you. We were excited for his embarkation on the next phase of his life, and at the same time hesitant to let him go for worry that his disease would continue to progress rather than abate. We were comforted to know an eating disorder therapist and dietitian worked in the health center at the school and would continue treatment with Jon. Also, the McCallum Place Eating Disorder Center was within 15 minutes of the campus if things got worse.

Jon had difficulty adjusting to SLU, some probably associated with the transition from high school to college and some related to his illness. He knew only one other student when he started, and a lot of students came from private parochial schools from the St. Louis and Chicago areas and tended to hang out in groups. He was hired at the sports arena and became involved in various organizations, one of which involved feeding the poor. Yes, *feeding*. One would think this was a wonderful organization for their college student to join. But it probably was not the best for a young man with anorexia whose desire is to control what others eat. These were the opportunities ED thrived on to give Jon an excuse to deny himself food.

During that freshman fall, Jon received treatment at the health center from a licensed psychologist, dietitian, and physician. With Jon's permission the dietitian, Rabia Rahman, communicated via email with me. However, over Thanksgiving break, we could tell things had continued to spiral downward regarding his weight, anxiety levels, and personality changes and knew we had to pursue more intensive treatment after he finished finals. We spoke with Jon about seeking treatment at McCallum during the second semester and threatened not to pay for school unless he went into the program. ED would have none of it. Crying, he promised he would fuel his body and exercise less. We continued to hold out hope and decided to wait until the end of winter break to negotiate with him, thinking, when he was home and done with the stresses of school, things would get better. We didn't make it that long.

I will never forget the call from Jon's physician while I was at Bible study two weeks after the fall break. She informed me that he was continuing to lose weight and exhibited elevated liver enzymes. She encouraged us to seek more intensive medical treatment. Sensing the urgency of her call, I left the women in Bible study as they prayed for Jon and our family and immediately drove to meet with her and Jon in St. Louis. He called me while I was on my way, begging me not to come. "I will be fine! You don't need to come!" he implored on the other end of the phone. What ensued during that visit was an intense crying and negotiating session at the clinic. I hated to see my son in such distress but knew ED had taken over and there was no turning back or getting cured without more intensive medical intervention. The weekly appointments with the therapist and dietitian were not going to be enough as Jon withered emotionally and physically. He continued to starve himself and exercise excessively. His life was at risk and he wasn't going to be able to continue school at SLU unless he sought more intensive treatment.

Behavioral Characteristics ("Anorexia Nervosa in Males", n.d.):

- Excessive dieting, fasting, restricted diet

- Food rituals

- Preoccupation with body building, weight lifting, or muscle toning

- Compulsive exercise

- Difficulty eating with others, lying about eating

- Frequently weighing self

- Preoccupation with food

- Focus on certain body parts; e.g., buttocks, thighs, stomach

- Disgust with body size or shape

- Distortion of body size; i.e., feels fat even though others tell him he is already very thin

Emotional and Mental Characteristics:

- Intense fear of becoming fat or gaining weight

- Depression

- Social isolation

- Strong need to be in control

- Rigid, inflexible thinking, "all or nothing"

- Decreased interest in sex or fears around sex

- Possible conflict over gender identity or sexual orientation

- Low sense of self-worth—uses weight as a measure of worth

- Difficulty expressing feelings

- Perfectionistic -- strives to be the neatest, thinnest, smartest, etc.

- Difficulty thinking clearly or concentrating

- Irritability, denial -- believes others are overreacting to his low weight or caloric restriction

- Insomnia

Physical Characteristics:

- Low body weight (15% or more below what is expected for age, height, activity level)

- Lack of energy, fatigue

- Muscular weakness

- Decreased balance, unsteady gait

- Lowered body temperature, blood pressure, pulse rate

- Tingling in hands and feet

- Thinning hair or hair loss

- Lanugo (downy growth of body hair)

- Heart arrhythmia

- Lowered testosterone levels

I contacted McCallum that day with a referral from SLU. Jon qualified for their Partial Hospitalization Program (PHP), and we were able to admit him upon his return in January. He would participate in a comprehensive program that included nutritional counseling by a registered dietitian, group therapy, and individual therapy by licensed psychologists on a daily basis for ten hours including meals. The choices were simple: attend treatment while at school at the clinic, pay for his schooling, or come home and attend treatment. Looking back, the choice was an easy one for ED. Being back at home under a watchful eye of parents AND undergo treatment? That would really stink for him. At least in St. Louis, ED could continue to exercise like a maniac and burn off any calories those tyrants would make him eat.

During that same visit, Debbie Barbeau, Assistant Dean of the Business School, met with us and was so helpful! She helped him rearrange his schedule so he could remain as a full-time student and participate in the McCallum program. I couldn't believe how kind she was to us. She didn't pry as we explained the circumstances to her. She saw a student that needed help and support and set out to do just that. Help. We left, feeling we hadn't been judged and with a new spring semester schedule. And I left feeling God's hand and renewed hope.

Over winter break, we could see Jon was really struggling. He had withdrawn from his friends. He barely met up with them and when he did, he came home early. He would tell us that he was going to eat with them. He didn't. But it was a great excuse for ED to avoid eating meals with us. Jon's friends were supportive but, understandably, became more distant and less inclusive as he withdrew physically and emotionally from them. When they were together, one friend, Hunter, would help me out by texting me answers to my questions about Jon's eating and activities. This was not the Jon he had known during high school and he did all he could to help. I was so thankful for him and his willingness to keep us informed. It was comforting to know Jon was safe with these old high school friends, hopefully enjoying their friendship, and not out exercising.

We continually discouraged Jon from exercise but that didn't stop him over the winter break. The second the house was empty, he would head out. We came home early one weekend evening around 10:00 as we often did at this point in his disease. They tell you not to allow your social life to revolve around the disease, but it is really difficult when you are worried. Anyway, Jon wasn't home, but his car was so my husband went out looking for him. He found him about a half mile from our home. Jon said he had lost his cell phone and had been looking for it. We knew he was out for another run. These blatant lies became more and more frequent and almost unbearable. This was not the son we knew. He had never been one to lie. When it pertained to exercise, eating, and socialization, we couldn't trust him to tell us the truth anymore. Unfortunately, he knew it and we knew it.

As I write, I wonder if the reader is thinking, "I can't believe you didn't pull him from school and admit him into a hospital!" It is not that easy. I think we were in denial as much as Jon was in the beginning. We thought that with a little support and monitoring of his meal plan, he would heal, regain weight, and things would return to normal. This thought process may be pretty common at the beginning. Remember, he had JUST started treatment and we had only one parental counseling session before he headed off to school. In truth, the disease progresses mentally, physically, and behaviorally. Patients need to qualify with certain criteria before admission into the programs. And, of course, insurance policies vary. Most patients don't get a diagnosis of anorexia nervosa and immediately get admitted into an inpatient program. There are outpatient, intensive outpatient, partial inpatient, and inpatient programs with different qualification criteria. And they ALL seem to have waiting lists for admission so you need to be proactive in seeking treatment early in the disease.

As Jon lost weight, ED was able to invade his brain more and more. His thought processes and behaviors became increasingly irrational. His lack of care for hygiene and dress were evident. It seemed he wore torn-up exercise clothes every day no matter what the occasion. As parents we tried to pick our battles. Clothing was usually not one of them. His daily focus was on calories and exercise and nothing else seemed to matter. ED would tell him things weren't that bad. He wasn't killing himself by exercising two and three times a day and should be proud that he wasn't fueling his body adequately. Look what control he had in his life! His parents and friends were crazy to be so concerned. ED is a liar and a manipulator and he fooled me more than once.

ED's control made Jon emotional. He cried when he felt he was disappointing us or his friends or when he was encouraged to seek more treatment. He wrote several letters to us during the course of his illness, apologizing for the hurt he caused us and thanking us for loving him. Those letters probably equaled the number of letters he wrote us rationalizing why he wasn't going to seek treatment, or to try to discharge himself from treatment. It was painful for us to see his hurt and shame. So what happens as a parent? You feel sorry for him. You feel guilty. You plead with him to eat, stop exercising, and follow treatment. I became emotional, crying in despair, and sometimes yelling out of anger. Those reactions were not helpful. I prayed.

Relying on hope and willpower, you negotiate and often give in to ED's demands. By doing so, however, you enable the disease to progress by giving its victim another chance to be consistent with treatment, fuel his body, and reduce the amount of exercise. I would go for a walk with him, hoping it would be enough and that he wouldn't sneak out later for a run. I hoped he was eating dinner like he said with friends, only to find out he hadn't. I made his favorite meals, hoping he could relax and enjoy one. As a loving parent, it is difficult to see that it is not a willpower issue and hopefulness won't turn into truth. Anorexia nervosa manifestation has various factors creating a torrential cycle that need to be addressed with professional help. My hope - our hope - had to be in God. We were not going to cure our son of this disease. He needed more.

The intensive program would turn things around, or at least stop the spiraling downward. We were sure of it. We knew he needed the intensive medical treatment. Even though he would go kicking and screaming, we were not going to give in this time. I think Jon felt the burden of overcoming anorexia was solely on his shoulders. He didn't deny he had the disease; he was in denial that it was life threatening and would require a team effort of family, dieticians, psychologists, physicians, and psychiatrists to battle it.

We traveled to St. Louis to attend family therapy. We visited often and tried to provide support over the phone but it wasn't enough. We wanted to support and encourage him, but often felt he perceived our words of encouragement as criticism. We were walking on eggshells around our son. He was defensive and on edge. We learned in therapy never to comment on his body. For instance, if we said, "You look good," he would hear, "You look fat." He always felt we were analyzing his every bite when, really, I was just thankful he was eating anything with us. He could have eaten 15 cupcakes for a meal and I wouldn't have cared! I say that in jest. The goal, of course, is to manage exercise and consume a healthy diet to provide enough fuel to maintain a healthy body and mind. But honestly, when your loved one is in this state, you desperately want them to eat and you don't care what they eat!

The program was wonderful but we had difficulty relating to others in the family sessions, and the distance made providing support challenging. What was difficult for us must have been 100 times more difficult for Jon. He spent 10 hours at the facility, with classes before and after. There were no other young men with anorexia to discuss challenges; he had a couple of friends at school; and he wasn't sharing with anyone that he was suffering from anorexia.

In addition, he was noncompliant with the treatment plan as he continued to exercise twice a day and skip group therapy sessions. He wasn't ready to accept and participate in treatment. I admit I didn't feel like our family's experience with the illness was similar to the young women in the group sessions. Many of them spoke disrespectfully to their parents. I remember one who pulled out a feeding tube to avoid a family session. I heard angry and snarky comments. Many attitudes just didn't seem the same as Jon's as I listened to their struggles and stories of their disease manifestations. Maybe it was just the gender difference that made it difficult to relate to the young women as a mother and son. Jon seemed more withdrawn and frustrated. He struggled with a lack of independence, wanted to feel like a normal student, and feared disappointing us. But again, I think maybe some parents and children believe they don't belong in this type of setting because they don't realize how sick they are. In fact, I learned from the Eating Recover Center in Denver, it is common to hear from patients in therapy comments such as "I don't belong here," "I'm not sick enough," "No one likes me here," "They lie to me," "Being here has helped me see that I have a problem. I can recover on my own now," "No one here understands me," "This place is making me worse," and "I am learning more about how to have an eating disorder here."

The distance contributed to our inability to provide adequate support and we focused on getting through the rest of his freshman year at college. Jon wanted to discharge himself the second week of February. However, the discharge would have been AMA, against medical advice, because of his low weight, and SLU would not allow him to return. The reality struck him enough to enable him to gain a few pounds that following week. He then discharged himself against medical recommendation, but it was not considered AMA. He was able to return to SLU. With lots of parental pressure, he reluctantly resumed visits with the SLU counselor and dietitian. These were inconsistent and we knew a battle would be on our hands when he returned from school with ED in full control.

COMING TO TERMS: Jon

The hardest thing for a man to do is ask for help. As a young man I looked up to my father and one trait he always exhibited was emotional strength. For example, he never sought help when dealing with problems or issues, whether it was in the garage or on the golf course. Some may call this stubbornness, but in my eyes this came across as the way a man should act, for it was also the way my grandfather and other men I looked up to acted. I am not trying to convey that this is the right way for a man to respond to problematic situations. After all, it is a common irritant to women, such as refusing to ask for directions when lost. But this is what I experienced growing up.

Coming to terms with my disease was the steepest climb on a road to recovery I would ever face, and it was difficult for me. Although I knew I was sick, I never accepted the extremity to which I was ill. I thought I could overcome it by myself with perseverance and determination. This is my journey.

I still remember the day I was diagnosed with the disease. My mom was concerned about my rapid weight loss and intense workout regimen. I had some hip pain so she took a look at it for me and noticed a lot of muscular atrophy. This added to her concern so she wanted to make sure my health was in order before I participated in my first full triathlon scheduled in a few weeks. My parents saw the workouts and restricted eating as part of my training, as did I. However, I lost eight pounds in the span of a month following my high school graduation. At the doctor's office, blood tests were run along with a general history and physical. Nothing came back abnormal from my blood tests; however, my doctor indicated that my heart rate was extremely low and he recommended getting an EKG to get a definitive sense of my heart's health. Later that day, we visited Shawnee Mission Medical Center where the first of many EKGs were run. The results indicated that my resting heart rate had a normal rhythm but had dropped to the low fifties. My doctor recommended that I not participate in the upcoming triathlon due to the possibility of cardiac arrest that might occur from the increased strain on the heart, and diagnosed me with anorexia nervosa. This news horrified my mom, for her father had died from a heart attack several years previously.

On the way home, I pleaded with my mom that I still needed to participate in the upcoming race due to the hard work and preparation I had put forth. I assured her that after the race everything would go back to "normal," that my eating habits would normalize, and my workout intensity would decline. She hesitantly agreed. I continued training up until the race. I completed the triathlon in just under three hours. I was very pleased with myself and this accomplishment. I thought, now I can resume life the way it was before. I was very wrong.

There was a two-month period in between my triathlon and my departure for college at Saint Louis University. Training intensity did not let up, and my weight, mental state, and health all continued to decline. My girlfriend and I agreed to end our long-term relationship due to the fact we would be attending different universities and did not want the stress and anxiety holding us back from enjoying our college experience. Today, when I look back, I think "what college experience?" and I chuckle to myself.

In August I departed for school with my mom and sister in the family SUV filled with all of my things. I was nervous and excited to start this new chapter of my life that everyone raves about. I immensely enjoyed high school so when it came to college I was quite skeptical whether life in college could match the hype. I was scheduled to continue therapy at an on-campus therapy center to please my parents, but I had every intention of enjoying life away from home, away from the worried eyes of mom and dad. Later that day, once I had all of my stuff unloaded and my mom and sister had departed, I was ready to start my life anew. I found out later that on that return journey, my sister and mom cried, not because their brother and son was going to school, but for fear for his life. I began school after losing another 5 pounds, totaling 13 pounds from my small frame since May.

Early on I got involved in the school community, joining numerous charitable, leadership, and cultural groups and organizations. I was part of the honors program in the business school and thus carried a difficult and full workload. I got a part-time job at the school's sports arena, helping the AV crew as an assistant to the camera man, which allowed me to sit courtside at all of the men's and women's basketball games.

I saw my parents approximately once every month, either by going home or having them come to town to visit. During their visits we would often talk about recovery and how I was doing both emotionally and physically. They could see that I was getting thinner and that my weight was continuing to decline. From my current mental state, I could not see that what I was doing was irrational. I started seeing a dietitian during my first semester at school, but often found myself lying when asked about my eating pattern in fear that my words would be communicated back to my parents. My social life during this time was minimal. I hung out with friends on my dorm floor, but never found myself "going out" much to enjoy all that St. Louis had to offer. I lost another three pounds.

That fall break I returned home. Little did I know I was in for a rude awakening as I found myself often on edge around food and working out. My parents were aware of my declining condition and started communicating more strongly about seeking solutions to my eating disorder. I found myself sneaking in workouts or runs while trying to keep my parents in the dark and naive about how serious the eating disorder had control of me. They cut off my gym membership, but that didn't stop me; I just enrolled at another. I was relieved when it was time to go back to school. I was happy to be leaving because it meant that I could continue my eating disorder in peace without the constant confrontation my family brought with them. However, the following semester my eating disorder would not be as uncontested as it was my first.

Back in St. Louis life continued as it had been. I was still a very involved freshman around campus and continued to make decent grades. My eating disorder did not allow me to exercise any less than two hours a day and I often went to the gym or ran twice a day. My breakfast regularly consisted of a Clif Bar, and lunch was a salad with lots of veggies and balsamic vinegar instead of salad dressing. I continued to see the therapist and dietitian, although little progress was made. I continued to work approximately 20-25 hours per week and often stayed in on the weekends to avoid social situations. At this point, I knew that the eating disorder had significant control over my actions and emotions, but I was personally too weak to fight it and what it had become.

Shortly after Thanksgiving break, my therapist, dietitian, and physician informed me I had lost too much weight and needed to seek more intensive treatment or I would not be able to continue my education at SLU. My mom came down that day to meet with them. It was a very emotional and stressful time and I hated the thought of having my time controlled by therapists and dietitians.

At Christmas break my parents had had enough of seeing this eating disorder control their son and presented me with three options. Either I pay for my school (my parents had generously accumulated saving in a 529 account for my education); I seek treatment at a local facility in Saint Louis, seven days a week; or I return home. Treatment would consist of day-long sessions starting at nine in the morning and running until five or six in the evening. Shocked by the ultimatum, I was discouraged, irritated, and distraught. I knew that I could not have the experience that I wanted in college going to this treatment center where I would be kept for ten hours a day, but who was I kidding. I wasn't having a true "college" experience to begin with, but my eating disorder didn't see it that way. Irrationally, I pleaded with my parents and asked that they give me just one more chance. I tried to convince them that things were improving in counseling and that I was truly getting better. They refuted my argument, noting that my weight and health had not improved and they had given me plenty of chances to combat the eating disorder on my own and now my ability to stay in school was being challenged. They said that they were not tired of me, their son, but of this life-sapping eating disorder that was taking their only son away from them. In the end I chose treatment. Not because I thought I could get better, but because I feared incurring the full load of student debt that would come with paying tuition without federal grants or loans.

My mom and I approached the Assistant Dean of the Business School. Because I was in the honors program, she was very comforting and understanding of the situation and I was allowed to enroll in adult education courses both early in the morning and late in the evening, something not normally allowed for undergraduates. I had to take a leave of absence from my job at the arena and discontinue my involvement in various on-campus student organizations since I would be unable to make meetings and scheduled activities. Life was about to change, but it wasn't for the better.

I arrived my first day at McCallum Place after the first of the year. I was introduced to my therapist and psychiatrist who I would be meeting with on a weekly basis during outpatient treatment. I was told that there were three meals a day with two snacks in between those meals. Our weight was taken first thing each morning. We were not allowed to exercise although I still did so each and every morning before both class and treatment. The days were filled with scheduled therapeutic classes, arts and crafts, and socializing. I was the only male patient in the facility and so I became friends with the women at the treatment center.

On my way back to my dorm each evening, I found myself pondering in disbelief that this is what my life had become. It was only ten short months ago that I couldn't imagine my life being any better as a responsible, accomplished high school student and athlete, and now I was a college student who couldn't even manage his own health adequately enough and needed to be sent to a treatment center for 50-60 hours a week for constant supervision. It was a low point, but it would only get lower.

I continued outpatient treatment at the facility for about five weeks. During that time, I continued to exercise in the morning and attend classes in the evening. My weight did not rise and my therapist knew the reason why, even though I would not openly tell her. I met with my psychiatrist weekly and our sessions often resulted in arguments over prescription medication that I refused to take.

Meal and snack-time would consistently go smoothly as I always finished my meal without much anxiety. I became friends with many of the patients and staff, but never felt comfortable and often found myself alone, being the only male patient in the facility. I wished I was home and to life before the disease.

A few weeks into treatment my mother came and visited me at the treatment center. She attended one of my group therapy classes and we conversed in the social area. We were not allowed to go out to lunch due to my low weight. During that visit, I broke down and pleaded that I be removed from this facility which I referred to as a jail; I would try harder to recover on my own with a therapist and dietitian to help me along the way. She began to cry, for it was her wish that her son be healthy and be able to live his life in a manner he wished, but she knew my train of thought was so irrational that removal from the treatment center might lead to death. Later that day she left.

I continued treatment at McCallum Place for two more weeks and shortly after removed myself from treatment after only a month. I continued to see a therapist and dietitian at school and let my eating disorder have total control. Soon the semester ended and I headed home for the summer.

PARTIAL INPATIENT TREATMENT: Lynn

Thankfully, I had an acquaintance in the neighborhood, Dr. Michelle Micsko, Licensed Psychologist and owner of InSight Counseling, a center for eating disorders. She happened to be driving by one cool evening to drop off some information for me in my mailbox. I was outside. She stopped and patiently listened to me as I spewed my frustrations and concerns regarding my son's health. She seemed to be the only one who really understood and I didn't really know her. I shared his treatment and his medical evaluation findings. His labs indicated elevated liver enzymes, continued bradycardia, and decreased white blood cell count. She urged me to seek more intensive treatment. She didn't mince words and said his systems were shutting down and if we didn't get him help he would die. This was the moment that seemed to slap me out of my "it will get better with just love and support" stupor. That my son might die kept resonating with me. If we didn't keep pushing to do something more, he would die. I am forever grateful for Dr. Michelle Micsko and for God who put her in my path that night. That truth, that reality shook me.

So our college student returned home. As with most families, there was a little bit of adjustment. There were some things that would upset any parent, let alone a parent of a son with anorexia. The behaviors associated with the disease were extremely evident. Being a fairly light sleeper, I would wake thinking I was hearing mice. Nope. It was Jon in the pantry getting a carefully measured half cup of cereal to sneak up to his room at midnight. Instead of being thankful that he ate, I would get upset waking to a dirty kitchen or pantry and feel frustrated that he couldn't eat with us. He proceeded to set up his waffle maker and air popper in his bathroom, of all places. Ahhhhh NO. I would wake to hear the front door squeak as he snuck out at 2 a.m. to go for a run. Our neighbor once passed him running in the middle of the night...wearing a weight belt. When we ate out, he insisted on choosing the restaurant and order a low calorie, fat-free meal and steal French fries off of our plates instead of ordering his own. He would down two to three glasses of water before sitting down to a meal. You might think, "He is going to a restaurant with you!" and "What a healthy kid!" Not so when you are a parent of a child who is starving himself. All you see are ED's behaviors and control. He ate pickles by the jar. He later told me he toasted Pop-Tarts after everyone went to bed so we would smell it and think he was eating and then throw it out the back door. These things all seem funny, normal, or kind of gross now; but at the time, they would either upset me or create worry.

We learned not to expect Jon to ask for treatment, and he certainly didn't enjoy attending sessions with the dietician and psychologist. One of the most effective tools we applied after treatment at McCallum and immediately when he returned home in May was the use of a contract. The contract allows you to establish rules for your household such as eating, setting goals coinciding with therapy, and improving communication. A contractual agreement helped us stay objective and act as a stepping stone to help Jon stay on track and seek further treatment which we knew he needed. A person has to want treatment to get over the addiction. If there is no desire, ED will fight like crazy. The contracts were also a necessity to keep our emotions in check and not battle over eating. In the end, Jon was suffering from the disease. We were there to support him. He had to make the choices associated with recovery.

Some of the contractual obligations Jon and we agreed to included attending appointments with his counselor and dietitian weekly, informing us when going to exercise, following the dietician's meal plan, ceasing taking food into his bedroom, not eating after 10 p.m., not drinking more than one glass of water with a meal, and returning to treatment immediately if his weight fell below a set goal. As the parents, we were not to discuss exercise or police his eating. As part of his therapy, I did prepare his meals according to his plan. Psychologically at this stage, it would have been impossible for him to prepare the meals according to the dietician's recommendations.

By that summer, it was easy to see how ED was destroying and taking his life. He was exercising incessantly, taking several naps throughout the day, sweating yet sensitive to cold. He took naps on the patio in 90-degree weather. He lacked muscle. His hair was thinning. I would hug him and feel his ribs. He was restless. After sitting still for 5-10 minutes he would jump up and occupy himself with activity or exercise while expressing feelings of unproductiveness at an unusual level. Eating was completely restricted and he continued to lose weight. He was socially isolated, cried often, didn't laugh, was lethargic, and just wasn't his humorous self. It was also during this period that he tearfully shared that he didn't want to return to Saint Louis University and wanted to transfer to another college. We certainly did not have a problem with this choice and supported him in his decision.

That's when we sought treatment at an inpatient center in Denver with Dr. Micsko's recommendation. Although Jon didn't qualify for full-time inpatient, he did qualify for a partial hospitalization program. Again, there was a waiting list. Although he tried to say "no" to treatment, he didn't have that option. Jon had broken every aspect of his contract with us. His systems were shutting down. He was not able to do this on his own, with just our help, or with outpatient therapy. We had a family intervention where he witnessed the pain and concern not only from me but his father and sister. Everyone was in tears, including his stoic father. If he chose not to go into treatment, we were prepared to seek Medical Guardianship. Finally, we convinced him to go into treatment at the Eating Recovery Center in Denver.

While he was on the waiting list, we took an extended family trip the grandparents had planned to celebrate their 50th wedding anniversary to Hawaii. We shared with them that Jon would be entering the Denver program and struggled with the decision to go; however, in the end we thought it would be best for our strained family relationship. ED had a hay day on that one. When he needed support the most at the height of his illness, it saddened me that no concern of his weight loss and health were openly expressed to Jon during the trip. The family knew he was suffering and going into treatment. However, Jon asked that minimal information be shared with others over the course of his illness so the grandparents really were the only ones who knew the severity. Everyone thought ED was so wonderful as he took orders to make breakfast one morning. Little did they know ED loves to control not only what the sufferer eats but also what others consume. This way of nurturing allowed Jon to deny himself food. He made sure he went for runs before anyone got up in the morning, continued restricting his intake, and was happy to excuse himself from the table to do dishes or supply any needed items. He continued to down water before meals, avoided any snacks and fats, and remained restless.

When we returned from the family vacation, Jon was admitted to the Eating Recovery Center in Denver at the end of July. Here he would live in an apartment with another young man who was also suffering from anorexia. Sadly, Jon learned later the disease took the young man's life. The program consisted of eleven hours of intensive therapy seven days a week. He would consult with a psychiatrist, therapist, dietician, nurse, internist, and chef. Treatment would also include yoga and art therapy. As a family, we would partake in family therapy sessions over the course of a three-day period. Their approach is ACT – Acceptance and Commitment Therapy. Accept your thoughts and feelings by acknowledging things are the way they are, you feel the way you feel; connect with your values by asking yourself what you can do that's truly meaningful or important; take effective committed action toward your value and when you stumble, get back up and carry on.

I think this was the first time that I got a full night's sleep in months. I felt that Jon was in a safe environment and receiving the treatment he required to get on a path of sustained recovery without the additional stress of school. When we participated a couple of weeks later in Family Days, we were educated and encouraged. However, Jon was not gaining weight, and in fact had lost weight. He was noncompliant regarding exercise and refused to take antianxiety medication as an adjunct to his treatment plan.

Ugh! However, we were confident that he had learned some coping tools to deal with his anxiety and was learning the proper ways to nourish himself, even though he was exercising when he returned to his apartment at night. To our dismay, Jon said he was discharging himself after a month in therapy. We did not pay for his flight home but hugged him when he arrived.

On a side note, one of the consistent frustrations we dealt with regarding medical treatment was Jon's age. He had turned 18 by the time he was diagnosed, which meant he was no longer considered a minor even though he was still a student and still covered under our medical insurance policy for which we paid the premiums, copays, and deductibles. What this meant, because of government mandated HIPPA guidelines, was that we were not allowed to receive medical updates or test results, attend consultations, or access records pertaining to his health unless he signed over permission with each caretaker. He could also discharge himself from treatment without our permission.

Thankfully, Jon didn't deny us permission to be privy to his medical treatment but there were a few times later in the disease when he required some coaxing. This was quite frustrating when our son's health and life were at stake. When we called for lab results, for instance, we were told that they couldn't share them with us because he was over 18. I found myself pointing out, sometimes with little patience, the line on the medical form where he had given us permission to access to his records. With that being said, we never crossed the line of private consultations with his therapists without him present and under their recommendation. The trust relationship with the therapist is an important one to honor throughout treatment.

PARTIAL INPATIENT TREATMENT: Jon

The summer of 2012 was the most unenjoyable summer I ever experienced. I was working as a server and taking two classes at the local community college. I came home that summer with the uncertainty that I wanted to return to Saint Louis University the following fall. Whether it was the chaotic schedule of treatment, work, and classes or the culture at a private school, I was unsure of the reason. However, when done with my first year of college I was often asked "did I love it at school?" and was unable to confidently say "yes." I mean in all honesty, how could I after the year I had just experienced?

I continued to exercise, and my difficulties with eating increased. I often found myself trying to trick my parents into thinking I had eaten breakfast after a workout by either toasting a Pop-Tart and then throwing it out into the woods, or making a breakfast sandwich and then instantly throwing it down the garbage disposal before my parents came down the stairs. The days I did eat breakfast it would be plain oatmeal or a slice of toast with jelly. All of this followed my two-hour workout each morning.

I continued to see a local therapist and dietitian per my parents' wishes. My weight started to decline yet again, and I began to tuck small weights and rocks under my shirts or in my pants during weigh-ins with the dietitian just so my weight would appear stagnant. With my lifestyle continuing to spiral out of control I soon found myself tucking five and ten pound weights in my jeans during my visits. Not once did I think this was rational and that I would be able to continue. However, my fear of returning to the treatment center was overbearing.

In July, my grandparents took their children and grandchildren on a once-in-a-lifetime trip to Hawaii for their 50th anniversary. I was very excited, for I had never visited the state of Hawaii although I had heard of the great island scenery and climate. A week before the trip I arrived home one night from work only to see my family all gathered in the family room with the television off. They each had a look of anguish and fear on their faces and so I knew the conversation about to take place was not going to be a positive one. My sister, dad, and mom each shared their fears and frustrations with my illness. My sister began crying as she spoke of her fear of losing her brother to this terrible illness. She missed my personality and the humor I once exhibited and wanted her "real" brother back.

I broke down in frustration and exhaustion. I was trying so hard to battle the eating disorder mentally, but for every step I took forward, it felt as though I would be dragged back and sink even deeper into the disorder. I knew my personality had changed. I knew I wasn't the person whom I was supposed to become, but I didn't know how I could fight any longer. I was tired, exhausted, and ready to give up. After I shared my thoughts, my parents told me that due to the life-threatening extent of my condition I had been accepted into one of the country's top eating disorder treatment centers in Denver, Colorado. I was to leave promptly after returning from our trip to Hawaii.

I was shocked, scared, and afraid. My worst fear had presented itself. I did not want to go back to the environment I had left a couple months ago. My parents told me that my choices were very bleak at this point. I was nearing the point of hospitalization and needed more extensive treatment than what was offered in Kansas City. I pleaded and begged them to change their minds, promising that I would work even harder to get back to a stage in which my health would not be so dire. They told me that this was the only solution and that if I refused, they would pursue legal action and place me in involuntary mental health treatment. They said that I could not beat this disorder in my current mental and physical state. I needed professionals and constant supervision to get all the tools necessary to beat this illness. Although sad and irate, I knew they were right. For over a year now I had been fighting the disease with no signs of improvement. I was left with little choice and, therefore, I agreed to go back into treatment.

Two weeks later we returned from Hawaii. I was to leave for Denver the following Thursday. As I mentally prepared myself for what I was about to experience, I still hoped that my parents would change their minds and allow me to stay. I resigned from my job and finished my summer classes. Soon after, I flew to Denver with my mom. In Denver, we drove to the treatment center where I was admitted into the facility for partial inpatient treatment. Feeling scared and alone, I told my mom goodbye as she left for the airport. I was introduced to my therapist, dietitian, and psychologist who I would be meeting with on a weekly basis. I met the patients with various types of eating disorders including bulimia and overeating. I continued to exercise and go for runs in the morning causing my weight to decline the first two weeks of treatment before it stabilized. I had lost fifteen percent of my body weight since the time of diagnosis and was 31 pounds underweight.

Around the third week I was there, I was scheduled to meet with my therapist and psychiatrist in a co-op meeting. They knew I had been exercising and were not blind to this sort behavior from their patients. They expressed their displeasure and tried to help me understand that medication may help ease the anxiety created by the eating disorder. I refused. I did not want to be on medication the rest of my life. Normal people did not have to take medication, why should I? I had never had to take a daily medication to function during my childhood and I was not about to start now. My parents called that night and pleaded that medication was an assistive tool to make recovery easier. They told me that I was running out of avenues in terms of recovery. If I continued to lose weight, I would be forced into hospitalization where a feeding tube may be required to avoid my organs shutting down. There they would have no choice but to legally take control of my treatment, since I was not in a physical or mental state to take care of myself. I was enraged. "How could they do this to me?" I thought.

I was lost, confused, and alone. I started to lose hope that I could recover from this disease. I hated the idea of spending another several months in this treatment facility. I was told that in order to regain mental clarity, I would need to reach about 90 percent of my true body weight. At my current weight, I could not see the light at the end of the tunnel and, therefore, had begun to lose hope that recovery was in the cards I had been dealt.

I did not plan to return to Saint Louis University for my second year of schooling. I started weighing my options for a transfer, evaluated different schools, and did some preliminary research during my time at the Eating Recovery Center. I soon began to tire of being at the center. I became frustrated and threatened to remove myself from recovery. After a little over three weeks at the treatment center, I discharged myself and bought a one-way ticket back to Kansas City. Very upset, my parents urged that I stay. Tired of feeling like a prisoner, I left and never looked back.

TREATMENT: Jon

During my almost three-year battle with anorexia, I visited two specialized treatment facilities, one in Denver and one in St. Louis. The programs were very similar to one another. I was required to arrive at the facility by eight or nine in the morning. The days ran until six or seven in the evening. Other than one other male, tenancy at these treatment facilities was female patients. The staff was also mainly female. This skewed tenancy reinforced the stereotype that eating disorders are a woman's disease and not one which men suffer. This concept played a significant role in my keeping the illness and its challenges to myself instead of sharing with others.

During my time at both treatment centers, I had the privilege of meeting one male staff member and one male patient. The male patient started suffering from the disease at a younger age than me. He appeared to be 14 when in actuality he was in his mid-20's and much older than I was. We were roommates during treatment in Denver and shared a two-bedroom apartment. We never got sentimental or shared too much detail about our suffering outside of treatment, but through basic conversation, I was able to see that our diseases stemmed from similar sources of athletics and perfectionism. A couple of months after I left Denver, I found out that he had passed away. It was a sad moment and an eye-opener as I saw what my fate could be.

Each day when I arrived at the facility, I was required to weigh-in, turn my phone over to the staff, and have my vitals recorded. Weigh-ins were conducted in a supervised room where I had to strip down to bare essentials and step on a scale to get an accurate reading. After re-dressing, my vitals were recorded twice, once standing and once sitting. In addition, my blood was drawn once a week to analyze organ function. My therapist and psychiatrist reviewed all of this information in order for them to assess my progress and recommend a course of treatment, but they never shared the results with me.

Each Friday I was required to choose my meals and snacks for the upcoming week. Meal changes were not allowed and sometimes my meal would be a surprise because I had forgotten what I ordered. All meals and snacks had similar caloric counts. Only non-caffeinated soda was allowed due to the effect caffeine has on heart rate and the false sense of fullness it provides, which is why it wasn't allowed during a meal. Meals were eaten in a family-style environment where conversation was strongly encouraged to remove some of the anxiety while eating. Sometimes games were brought to the table to create conversation and distract our minds from the meal in front of us. Everyone was required to stay seated during meals and finish everything on their plate. By everything, I mean "EVERYTHING." Normally, I never had trouble finishing my meals. One exception was when I decided to try a beef entrée. The beef was good except for the solidified fat. As anyone would do, I carved away the fat and gristle only to be shocked when I was required to consume them before leaving the table. That was only time I truly had a hard time finishing my meal.

In between meals, snacks, and therapy and psychiatrist appointments, we attended therapeutic classes designed to help alleviate the stress and anxiety that we associated with food. The classes often involved everyone sitting in a circle and taking turns sharing thoughts. The goal was to find the root of what led to restrictive eating and exercising obsessively. In addition to therapeutic classes, we engaged in classes such as yoga and art and crafts. I also had free time in which I could read, talk, or surf the internet on censored computers and laptops. During my free time I found myself in the arts and crafts room working on different projects for friends and family. This was highly unusual, as I was not creative and did not usually enjoy doing crafts. However, arts and crafts allowed me to keep my mind occupied and away from thoughts associated with the eating disorder. It kept my hands busy and allowed me to express some of the apologetic emotions I felt towards my family. It was keeping busy that really helped me.

As I noted before, I was required to turn in my phone for the sole purpose of censorship. If you struggle with an eating disorder, taking your phone and the daily routine of treatment may sound like hell. It is a challenge, one that I was not willing to face. I was not strong enough to stick with the process and fulfill the course of treatment. It made my eating disorder very unhappy to be cooped up in a facility five to seven days a week and constantly monitored; however, I DO believe that it helped during my short times there. I learned several coping mechanisms to deal with the anxiety food provoked. This may come across hypocritical, since I pulled myself out of both treatment facilities after short stints. I am no way saying that my experience and actions are ones that patients with eating disorders should follow. What is the saying I am looking for? "Don't do as I do, but do as I teach." Easier said than done, right?

I made some friendships at these facilities as well. Although they were mainly women, it was helpful to have friends experiencing similar issues. Treatment is tough, to say the very least. One should be ready to give it 110 percent. While I am not a role model for the ideal patient in treatment, it helped many of the friends I made. Sadly, some have passed away and some are still struggling, but many have returned to living healthy and fulfilling lives free from the eating disorder. I would encourage you, if you are struggling, to seek help. Whether it is outpatient or in-patient treatment, every bit helps. No one is too big for help.

ROAD TO RECOVERY: Lynn

When he returned from Denver without completing the program, we again implemented the contracts, which he now abided by more consistently. We didn't want to repeat the mistake of trying to provide support over a distance during treatment so we required him to stay home for the fall semester of college. However, we did allow him to enroll in a couple of courses at the local junior college to apply toward his degree. During this time, he went to therapy sessions at Insight Therapy owned by Dr. Micsko who had encouraged us to get him into more intensive treatment in Denver. To avoid a conflict of interest, Jon developed a trusting relationship with another therapist, Kirsten Oelklaus, LSCSW and dietitian, Katy Harvey, MS, RD, LD. He began investing in the stock market to fill his time, completed crossword puzzle after crossword puzzle to occupy his mind and, yes, exercised. We didn't buy him a gym membership so he purchased one on his own. Remember, these are their choices. We can't control but we did not enable either. We also participated in therapy with a different psychologist so as not to undermine the trust relationship he had with Kirsten.

By the end of the semester, he had gained enough weight to allow us to feel we could trust him to follow through with treatment while he was 40 minutes away at college. However, he was not back to the 90th percentile that we had hoped. This, by the way, was the magic number that therapists encourage a patient to achieve. Mind function, physical health, and rationalization ability improve dramatically at this healthier weight.

He enrolled at KU for spring and started out well. We were quite hopeful as he moved in with a friend from his childhood, Dylan. He lived with his girlfriend at the time. Jon agreed to continue counseling with his current therapist in the area and began seeing a dietician closer to school. He got a job working as a barista in a coffee shop. At first he continued with therapy, but soon visits became inconsistent and nonexistent. Jon reverted to his restrictive eating, isolation, overzealous exercise regimen, and the other behaviors that accompanied him before his treatment in Denver. He was religiously eating a half dozen yogurts, sushi, protein bars, protein shakes, and wheat puffs for meals. He walked to and from school, rain or snow, which was a couple of miles away. He would never eat dinner with his roommates. The eating disorder characteristics caused friction between them resulting in a parting of the ways at the end of the academic year. The parting really saddened us and his lifelong friend.

Because he was under contract with us, he was forced to either return to rehab or pay for his own living expenses. He chose to pay rent and live at school over the summer. He found a room in a house with women who were students but total strangers. Although the location was right next to the school, we were very uncomfortable with the stranger living situation.

This tough love approach was extremely difficult for my husband and me but we were not willing to enable ED. Money tended to speak loudly to Jon so we held firm and chose to make sure we kept in touch frequently throughout the weeks. We knew we needed to stay strong but were unsure what result would come out of it. Constantly, in the back of my mind, I remembered reading that to improve the chances of success in treatment of anorexia nervosa there was a three-year window if it was caught early. Jon was into his third year. During that spring, he started seeing a dietitian in the area but continued to avoid therapy sessions back in Kansas City.

Like most college young men, I imagine, he didn't exactly encourage our visits. Whenever we drove out to visit and take him out for lunch or dinner, which I am sure he looked forward to with eager anticipation, we would see plain yogurt, canned green and refried beans, oatmeal, protein powder jars, and protein bar wrappers. He didn't enjoy our visits and honestly, my heart sank each time. I longed for the day when we would be able to take him and his roomies out for dinner and talk about school, sports, and parties.

However, toward the end of this summer and into the fall, we began to see a change in Jon. He pledged the Christian fraternity, Beta Upsilon Chi, or BYX, in the spring and made some good friendships. His weight loss appeared to have stopped and something began changing in his attitude. He wasn't inviting us out to dinner yet, but he wasn't avoiding meals or spending time with us when we invited him. We helped him move in with a classmate and his friend that fall and then into an apartment on his own the following fall where he completed his last semester of college, graduating in three years. Meanwhile, he worked at a job he really enjoyed as a waiter in the university's "upscale" café and seemed to be balancing his health, school, work, and social life.

As Jon will tell you, each person is different in the way they will respond to their disease. We agree with him that he had to hit rock bottom before he could pick himself up. Whether it was a turning point to lose a lifelong friend, being cut off financially, or a revelation that summer, I will let him explain, I don't really care! By the grace of God, somewhere there was a turning point that started him on the road back to us, back to his friends and family, and most importantly back to himself.

ROAD TO RECOVERY: Jon

Arriving back in Kansas City from Denver, I continued life as it was before. I continued to see the same therapist and dietitian I had been seeing in Overland Park and continued to exercise. I got a job as a server and enrolled to take six credit hours at the local community college. My parents continued to show displeasure and frustration with my eating disorder as it was obvious I was showing minimal effort to recover. At this point, I had become content with my situation and what life was to look like going forward. I was tired of trying to beat this disease and was slowly awaiting death. Although I knew it would not happen soon, eventually the stress that I was putting on my organs and muscles would lead to the inevitable. In November, I enrolled at the University of Kansas since going out of state as a transfer student was incredibly expensive. I organized a living situation with a good friend of mine from high school who was living with his girlfriend in a three-bedroom house. I was ready to start the last chapter of my life.

In January I started school at the University of Kansas. I continued to see my therapist and dietitian in Overland Park, although I often created excuses not to attend sessions. I later transferred to a dietitian closer to college. My eating habits continued to be strange, such as consuming excessive amounts of yogurt and bran crackers, and my intense exercise continued. It was the same story in a new location. I did well in school and ended my first semester with a 3.3 GPA. That summer I decided to stay in Lawrence to avoid my parents back at home. I worked as a barista at a local coffee shop, but was soon let go due to financial difficulties by the mom and pop store. I lived in a house just off campus with three women whom I had never before met. They were in need of an extra roommate to help cover rent and I was in need of a place to live. I soon was selected to be a Junior Research Assistant for the Center of Policy and Research at the university. It was a unique opportunity that provided employment for the rest of the summer.

During this summer I experienced my lowest point of recovery. One particular day I considered going against my morals I was raised with and almost stole. Because of the control the disease exerted on every aspect of my life, my unwillingness to follow through with treatment, and my decision to not return home and to live on my own, my parents had stopped funding my living expenses. Working part-time at the coffee shop, my income was not exactly booming so I was struggling as money left my bank account at a more rapid pace than ever before. You see, growing up, I had always been a saver. My parents often called me cheap, but I preferred the term frugal, so seeing more money going out than coming in alarmed me. The eating disorder's irrational thought process took over. I found myself considering stealing bran crisps. This disease had me thinking I should steal some lousy, tasteless, menial bran crackers. All I could think was, "This is not who I am. This is not who God wants me to be." I had always taken pride in my morals, character, and religious upbringing and now I was going against all of those things, thanks to this life-controlling disease. This was when I knew something needed to change. It wasn't until that moment that the true desire to change really sunk in.

For two years, my parents and sister had wanted me to get better. They supported me and often broke down to me, praying that I would have a change of heart and embark on recovery. I responded with all the correct words, lies, and phrases to temporarily ease their pain and suffering, but they knew I didn't mean it. It wasn't until I hit rock bottom that the switch was flipped; the flip that sparked the desire that so many wanted for me. I decided to take control myself.

I was re-energized to restart recovery. I didn't care what it was going to take. I was not going to let myself continue being what this eating disorder had turned me into. I had never been a quitter and I was certainly not going to start now. I had several dietitians during my recovery and each one always targeted ninety percent of a healthy body weight to get my mind functioning rationally once again. This is the goal that I set for myself.

The process of recovery started with what I knew best at the time, counting calories. I began binging on Pop-Tarts in order to take in the calories in smaller quantities, justifying to myself why it would be okay to eat one more. At my peak, I was consuming a box of Pop-Tarts a night. This went on for the rest of the summer. To this day, I cannot eat a Pop-Tart. I guess I ruined that for me. After the Pop-Tart craze started, I found myself eating raw brownie mix. I know, all of this stuff is weird, but I did what I had to do to put on the weight I needed to regain control of my mind and body. I am not suggesting that the way I gained my weight back was proper or would be suggested by a professional dietitian, but I had one phrase in my mind the entire time, and that was "just eat." I didn't care how I did it. I knew I would be able to regain normal eating patterns later after I was thinking properly and could battle this disease.

Ironically, my fear was always that gaining this much weight back so drastically would make me "blob-like." I was sure that humans were not supposed to gain weight back this fast and still be the athletic specimen I desired to be. It was the biggest struggle I dealt with in my mind. As you know, the first several pounds I gained back were not in the healthiest of ways. Even so, I did not look like a blob after gaining the weight back that quickly. Slowly but surely, I started winning back pound after pound. I feared for so long that the weight that came back would be in the form of body fat, but I was at the point of not caring anymore. Slowly my weight rose and I saw that the weight gain was not making me fat, but helping me become more energized and alive. My personality started to shine through the darkness as pound by pound, I got closer and closer to my ideal body weight. I continued to eat a box of Pop-Tarts a day and upped my food quantity for the rest of that summer. In the fall I continued at school, living with a friend whom I had met in one of my geography classes the previous semester. I had gained eight pounds back.

During the fall of 2015 I continued to increase my quantity of food. As my weight increased, I incorporated more diversity into my diet. I stopped eating plain oatmeal and started to challenge myself at the grocery store. My parents could see the progress I was making as I recovered more and more of my personality each day. I took baby steps, and once I reached 90 percent of my ideal body weight, my mental clarity started to come back and I could see how disillusioned I had been during the low points of my illness. I knew that the battle with my eating disorder was still not won, but for the first time in two years, I had the upper hand.

Over the next semester I focused on balancing work, recovery, school, and social activities at the University of Kansas. I have never been a huge fan of alcohol so making friends with a year and a half left in college was difficult. Luckily, I found Beta Upsilon Chi, a Christian-oriented fraternity, on campus. I pledged that spring semester, knowing I had only a year left of school before graduation. Over the next year, between work, school, and life at the fraternity, I was finally, truly experiencing life at college.

RELATIONSHIPS: Jon

One of the greatest impacts that the eating disorder had was on my relationships. Combining an eating disorder that promotes isolation with the transition to college is a recipe for disaster. I don't wish to share my relationship struggles so you may feel sorry for me. No. I want to share them with you so you may be able to battle your eating disorder and not let it affect your friends and family to the extent that I let mine do so.

My sister, Bailey, and I grew up together like two peas in pod. Just sixteen months apart, we always found each other in similar stages of our lives and so it was easy for us to share in life's learning curves. Although we didn't have the "always have to be together" type of relationship, we had a weird bond that when we got together, it was like we just saw each yesterday. I love my relationship with my sister. We have independent lives and are able to enjoy each other's company when we are together. During my illness, Bailey was away at school in Fort Worth at Texas Christian University. I often gave her a hard time for not coming home frequently enough, but today I think I am glad it was that way. I am not sure how my eating disorder would have changed our relationship, but I don't think it would have been for the better. During the time that I, my sister, and my eating disorder were together I could see frustration within my tolerant sister. She was tired of seeing my personality, which was so vibrant, constricted by the eating disorder. She saw me isolate myself and avoid situations with my friends. Bailey was often part of confrontations my parents would have with me regarding the severity of my eating disorder. Unlike my parents, she would speak timidly of her concerns. Today, I consider Bailey one of my closest friends. I am very proud of both her and her accomplishments. I cannot imagine the impact that my disorder might have had on our relationship if she hadn't been so far away. However, I am glad that I never had to find out.

The tension with my parents throughout my eating disorder was tumultuous to say the least. Every day was a new battle, one in which the eating disorder would try everything in its power to stay in control. My parents exhausted every option they had when trying to solve the riddle that confronted us. They offered everlasting support and undying love, never judging me or abandoning me during recovery. Although our relationship may have changed, it was not for the worse. Sure we fought more often than before, but my mom and I would have long talks discussing relationships, life, and education. Those talks helped me develop my own thoughtful opinions on matters such as politics, finance, and social issues. It helped me mature and become the man I am today. My dad and I had similar talks while throwing the football in the front yard. As a result, I saw my relationships with both my mom and dad deepen and become what they are today. During the illness, however, my parents distrusted me. The journey to recover their trust was not long, but it did take time. I hold so much appreciation for the solidarity of my family and its bedrock foundation. I wish every child, teen, and young adult could be blessed with the family foundation that I have. I consider myself extremely lucky and blessed for the situation that God put me in.

Information was shared with my grandparents; however, my aunts, uncles, and cousins had little knowledge of my eating disorder and its severity. I am positive that they would have shared the same love, compassion, and support my parents had, but at the time I preferred that as few people as possible knew the extent to which my health was suffering. I was embarrassed and ashamed. I often feared others knowing and judging me as the "kid with an eating disorder." There was also the inability of others to understand. The answer to an eating disorder is to "just eat," but the implementation is not that simple. Explaining the depth and roots of the issue were not something I was prepared to share.

There is one situation, however, that I can specifically recall that affected my relationship with my extended family. My dad's side of the family was in Hawaii for the trip prior to my admittance to treatment in Denver. During the trip, I was weak, emotionless, and just not the kid I used to be. My Uncle Tom, who is also my godfather, lives in California and was on the trip. I never got to see my uncle as much I wished. I always thought he was the "coolest" guy and we would often bump our sarcastic senses of humor off each other at family events and get-togethers. During the trip, however, my sense of humor was non-existent and I found my sarcasm could easily be misconstrued. This was the case during a joking encounter with my uncle that trip which led to a never-before-seen, stern expression of frustration. During my treatment in Denver, I called Uncle Tom and explained the situation. He had no idea and was astonished when I told him the extremity to which I was suffering. He was so proud of me for seeking treatment and was often lost for words during our conversation. Of course, there was no reason for him to be proud of me since I sought treatment based on an ultimatum and not by choice. Since my recovery, our relationship is back to normal.

My friendships were the most significantly impacted tier of relationships during my eating disorder. In high school, I had a bountiful supply of friends. Due to my friendly and humorous personality, it was easy for me to be comfortable around the majority of my classmates. During the transition from high school to college, I saw most of my friends become consumed with life at college; relationships were strained and became non-existent, which is probably typical and totally normal when separated by the distance between schools. However, combining natural occurrences with the isolation that my eating disorder promoted created even greater strain on those relationships. When get-togethers during college breaks were organized, I often found myself leaving early or not going so I could be alone and not face the anxiety that the eating disorder created in social situations. I am saddened when I think about the relationships my eating disorder ruined. Some I was able to repair, but not to the extent to which I wish they could be. I met a group of guys through my Christian Fraternity, BYX, at the University of Kansas. Two, Brian and Josh, are currently roommates and good friends of mine. This group of guys has become my core group of friends; however, I find our bond is not as deep as the one I had with the high school group which I blame on the time I lost while in treatment, transferring schools, and through isolation. I still am working on my relationships with friends, family, and co-workers on a daily basis and understand that time is the key component when building relationships. I am sure that ten years from now, I will look back and wonder what I was so worried about, but as of right now this is where my relationships lie.

My dog, Champ, is one of the most prosperous relationships I have had since my recovery. I adopted Champ from the humane society shortly after the summer of 2013, the summer I gained back a significant amount of weight and was nearing the point of full recovery. He is a dark brown beagle/pug mix (puggle) and weighs about 25 to 30 pounds. Champ's name is symbolic for me and is also a nickname that my dad often called me. I had always wanted a dog of my own, but knew during my disease that I could not take care of another living creature, much less take care of myself. When I adopted Champ he was six years old and had been rescued from abuse and inhumane treatment. He had been transferred all over western Kansas, and Lawrence was his last shelter before he would be considered unadoptable and euthanized. I like to think that we "saved" each other. The first day that I had Champ, it felt like we had been together since he was a puppy. He sat by me on the way home from the humane society licking my face.

A couple of weeks later, I found out that Champ had severe anxiety (ironic, I know), was afraid of pole-shaped objects (probably from the abuse he suffered), and was petrified of crates. As of today, all of those issues have drastically improved. Champ is now nine years old and the best dog I could possibly have asked for. My family adores him and I hope that if he could speak, he would me tell me that I was a savior in his life as he was in mine. If you ask my roommates, they can certify we are each other's best friends.

LIFE TODAY: Lynn

Today, Jon is a college graduate with a job that he loves. He has roommates that he likes to hang with in a house that he proudly purchased on his own after a year of working. Although we reimbursed him after seeing sustained health maintenance, he also invested well the fall he stayed at home. He apologized to those he hurt and his family and friends have forgiven him, including those high school friends who reached out to a friend they saw needing help and the elementary school roommate. He has reconnected with those who were closest to him and provided support over the years. As a mother, I will always be grateful to Hunter, Morgan, and Dylan who reached out and tried to help.

It has been five years since his diagnosis. His lowest weight was 74 percent less than what it is now – fit, healthy and muscular. He shares his story openly and honestly in the hope of helping other young men suffering from this disease to come forward and seek treatment before it is too late.

We have a wonderful relationship that includes healthy exercise and going out for meals together. He may not ever again want what used to be his favorite meal, chicken parmesan or shrimp fettucine with Caesar salad and garlic bread, but I can live with that. It isn't that he can't consume them individually, but all together it provokes excessive anxiety. However, in retrospect, this is a healthier choice, one that I could learn. He eats very healthily but doesn't restrict his diet. He enjoys variety again. For example, he will eat oatmeal but isn't afraid to add fruit or even a little sugar to it. The key is eating a healthy diet at a level high enough to fuel his activity so that he remains at a healthy weight.

I knew he was on his way to renewed health when he handed me the weights he used to improve the scale reading at the dietitian's office. I loved when he called me and shared that he had made a recipe with the full amount of cheese, and when he had returned from trips with friends for ice cream. These everyday things mean little to someone who hasn't dealt with anxiety related to food. To me? I know how hard Jon has worked to overcome anorexia nervosa so these phone calls make me rejoice as he continues to achieve success. Success that makes him happy and allows him to feel "normal," in his words. His personality has returned along with his witty humor and beautiful smile.

Is everything roses? No. I can see at times that he struggles to engage in social situations but is at ease when he does. He needs to follow his schedule and gets a little stressed when it gets knocked out of whack. And he does have difficulty remaining idle and always seems to be working on a project or volunteering. Can't all of us say we are a work in progress? Like most moms, I wish he ate a few more fruits and veggies to balance the protein. But yes! It did get better for us. He eats a healthy diet and exercises in a healthy manner. As long as he is fueling his body to maintain his weight, we are thrilled and no longer worry about him. It's been a long race, but we can see the finish line. We hope the same success holds true for you.

As Jon, I, and the experts have pointed out, there are many factors that play a role in the perfect storm of anorexia nervosa. Each case is unique and needs to be treated as such. As I reflect on those years and what helped us through the fire, I can summarize the following points from our experience:

First and foremost, our faith in God. Jon volunteered throughout his years of suffering in our church coffee shop, interacting with people when otherwise he would probably have chosen to isolate himself. He often went to the altar to pray for healing. He and I chose to surrender our lives to Christ during that time and we renewed our baptism by immersion. He joined the BYX Christian fraternity at the university and made some wonderful friends who he continues to hang with socially.

I was part of a Bible study in my neighborhood that was full of women whose hearts were after Christ. They continued to pray for me and my family week after week when I felt so alone. It was someplace I felt safe from gossip and protected. I still get tears in my eyes when I think of my friend, Allison, who prayed out loud for Christ to let me see that I was a loving mother when I was feeling like a horrible one unable to help my son. Another close Christian friend, Lianne, would walk with me, listen, support, and hug me. I laugh now when I think how many times she probably left me thinking, "Thank God I am not her!" My friend, Annie, was always there, as well, to lend a shoulder when needed. I truly surrendered to the power of Christ's healing during this time. I have learned to pray and be thankful each and every day. He brought me. He brought our family. He brought Jon through this fire with a renewed faith and trust in Him and His power.

Secondly, contracts! They will help keep you focused on support and help guide your loved one to the treatment he requires. I won't lie. I was not perfect. I cried. I pleaded. I raised my voice at times. I was sometimes critical and not always a wonderful supportive mother! But contracts allow you to hold strong against ED and keep everyone pointed in the right direction of healing. But you must be willing to do your part as well by holding firm to criteria you have established. Don't allow yourself to be manipulated by ED.

Third, separate ED and your son. My son told me he didn't like it when I referred to ED but I needed to separate the two to control my frustration. ED changes your loved one. It takes over his mind and body. I found it helpful to separate the two so I could stay focused on the love for my son.

Fourth, read and listen. The websites shared in this book are so helpful in understanding the disease and providing guidance for support and treatment. Seek out reputable professionals who have experience in eating disorders, listen, and follow through. This includes attending counseling sessions as a family. This disease affects your loved one the most, of course, but it also touches all of those who care about him.

LIFE TODAY: Jon

While I was in several different treatment programs during my time with the eating disorder, there was always one common idea that was conveyed to me as I looked for the finish line. I was told that "normalcy" would come and that my life would go back to what I thought "normal" was. I know you are looking for comfort and support so I hope not to scare you, but I still face challenges day in and day out. It is this reality that brings the question to mind, "Am I truly cured?"

After recovery, I decided to help write an article for the local newspaper, The Kansas City Star, authored by Jim Fussell (2013), to spread awareness of eating disorders in male sufferers. I received numerous phone calls asking for advice for sufferers and receiving support for my struggles. Even after the article was published, I was still not at ease with what I had gone through. I struggled with the concept that something commonly misunderstood as a "women's disease" ruined three years of my life. I was filled with hypocrisy regarding my eating disorder. Sure I gained almost 40 pounds back and had resumed normal trains of thought, toned down my workout regime, and eliminated fears of certain types of food, but the thought was still lurking. When I approached a meal, I still found myself thinking more than I used to. When food was approaching, I could feel the wheels starting to turn in my head, not provoking extreme anxiety like before, but still diligently thinking through what I was consuming.

Along with the thoughts, I also struggled with my personality. With the eating disorder controlling my personality for so long, I had forgotten who I was. I struggle with the idea that this is who I really was meant to become. Is this me? Or is the result a man influenced by a past eating disorder? During my childhood and teenage years, I had a vibrant sense of humor and was seen as the "energy" in the room. Today, I find myself less flexible and more rigid with my responsibilities and tasks. I still am able to display that sense of humor, but it doesn't come as easily as it once did. After struggling with an eating disorder during such a critical time in my life, I wonder if this is who I was supposed to be today. Is my change actually a result of maturity or a result of not being able to live out a crucial time in my life where I was able to "step out on my own" and live independently. This is just one question that I consistently struggle with and one that I do not think I will ever answer.

You might think, "Will I ever have a healthy relationship with food?" During recovery, this question seems like the most difficult to answer. While in Denver, I told my therapist that my goal was to have a burger and fries with my Dad at a Kansas favorite, Johnny's Tavern. I longed for the times pre-disease when my Dad and I went to the tavern after soccer practice to order their special, two-for-one burgers. This memory seemed so distant and impossible to relive that although I shared this goal with my therapist, I didn't believe it myself. However, I do want to share that the goal is not impossible, but highly probable. It is remarkable the kind of changes that take effect once your mind is able to function properly. You are able to regain your common sense and rational thought.

Would I say that I am still as careless with what I eat as I was pre-disease? That question, again, is tough to answer. Today, I am a lot more cautious with what I put in my body. I do not restrict the quantity of food that I put into my body, but I do find myself putting a lot more thought behind my food choices than I once did. It is my opinion that this is both an effect of my affinity for fitness and health and the lasting effects of recovery. During recovery, as you regain your weight, you are required to put extensive thought into your food choices to make sure that you are incorporating all categories of food (carbohydrates, proteins, and fats). For me, my fear was consuming fats. As a result, I would find myself having to think "Does my meal contain any fat? If not, how can I add some so that my meal will be balanced?" Having this thought process three times a day for 365 days a year can really stick with a person.

The most satisfying feeling that I have experienced regarding my relationship with food is that I no longer fear certain foods. As I shared before, my fear was primarily of fats. I feared consuming any sort of fat. I was aware of its importance, but was unable to think clearly about the fact that I need to be consuming it in my diet. Today, I can definitely state that I do not fear fat any longer.

When I had the eating disorder, I worked out excessively and felt drained both physically and mentally. Enjoying the activities I once did was no longer easy as my mind focused on food and caloric intake. I wasn't able to exhibit the same enthusiasm and energy I once had which diminished my quality of life. For example, I volunteered for numerous events, groups, and activities in college. However, I was never able to engage enough to enjoy the experiences. The eating disorder masked the experience by filling my mind with anxieties around food and social situations. My diminished quality of life during these three years is the one thing that haunts me the most.

Today, I still have difficulty comprehending the damage my eating disorder had on my relationships with friends and the experiences I missed out on during college. However, I have come to terms with my past experiences and have decided to learn from them rather than dwell on them. My friends say I am very responsible and always working on something whether it is volunteering, business, or fixing things around the house. Although this may stem from an inability to relax, I do what I value, which makes me feel alive.

Now, I volunteer weekly at both my church and as a recreational sport coach. I love working with the young kids and helping them learn something new while staying active in the process. I am able to express the enthusiasm and energy that I once had each and every practice and game which, in itself, is a great feeling but especially when you are able to bring a smile to a child's face. At church, greeting weekly patrons and putting a morning smile on their face makes every Sunday great. These might come across as silly and minor things, but they make a world of difference to someone who knows what life is like when you had the inability to express emotions.

Not knowing how to make a sick child better is a parent's worst fear and one that no parent should have to go through. Unfortunately, God made the world one of challenges, with disease being one of them. Standing strong, supporting the suffering, and believing that God has a plan are three of the most important things you can do as a parent.

As a child who made two parents go down the long road of his recovery, I have a sense of how much pain my illness caused them. For about a year after healing, I frequently found myself feeling guilty for all the pain, money, and suffering I caused my parents. They reassured me week after week, that when it comes to their children, money is no object. However, my cost-conscious mind would not let the guilt go. Eventually, the feelings that plagued me subsided with the vast amounts of reassurance my parents offered. I guess when you are told something often enough, eventually it sticks.

Today, my parents are both happily retired and enjoy having their kids working as professionals nearby. I would say that based on what I have seen, no parenting experience or journey is perfect or easy, but staying with it and offering support, advice, and help will lead to healing. Today our relationship is renewed and better than ever. We are able to enjoy mealtimes and talk about favorite foods, as well as go to restaurants without having to deal with food as interference, including two-for-one burgers at Johnny's with my dad.

I often joked with my dad about his receding hair line during my childhood. I saw his hair grow drastically thinner in those two and half years I suffered from anorexia. This was probably due to the stress I caused. However, post-illness, I have seen his hair grow back, thicker and denser than I can remember. It is, honestly, the strangest thing. Might also be the retirement, who knows?

What can I suggest to someone who is dealing with a child or loved one struggling with an eating disorder? Patience is the key to all healing. The healing will not happen overnight. It is a process of trial and error, encouragement and support. One who suffers from an eating disorder, I believe, needs to hit rock bottom before he or she wants to recover. I cannot stress that one word enough, "wants." The sufferer has to want to get better in order for him or her to do so. You, as a parent, family member, or friend cannot make the disease-stricken person recover. Anorexia is not like cancer or the flu, it is an action-driven disease and there is no medicine in the world that can alone cure the disease.

DR. MICHELLE MICSKO'S PERSPECTIVE

I have waged war with a formidable opponent for twenty-eight years. At times he has won. Those were dark days. He almost took away from me what I love to do many times. I have been able to stay in the fight against my nemesis and today I feel stronger against him than I ever have. My opponent is not an athletic or political rival, because if you lose in those battles, you come in second. If you lose to my opponent, you die. My opponent is cunning, sharp and knows his prey better than anyone because he knows their every thought. My opponent is the same beast with which Jon Sestak and his family found themselves in the fight of their life. Our mutual nemesis is an Eating Disorder. I fight against him in my office every day, but I get to go home and try to have an evening and weekend without him. Jon and his family didn't have that luxury. They couldn't escape for breaks because they lived with him twenty-four hours a day, seven days a week, for years.

ED VS. THE GOOD GUYS

I look at treatment much like a war. It is a long, long fight. I always tell families they are in for a marathon, not a sprint. It is a calculated battle with well-thought moves both on the eating disorder's part and on the part of the good guys, the recovery team. The recovery team consists of the healthy part of the individual struggling with the eating disorder, their family, and the treatment team usually comprised of a psychologist, dietician, physician, family therapist, and often a psychiatrist and eating disorders therapy group. I see each step in recovery as a battle in the long war. Sometimes the eating disorder wins the battle and sometimes the good guys win. Unfortunately, both sides are fighting very hard to win.

A SYMPTOM IS NOT A LIE

I will call the eating disorder, "Ed". Professionally, we give the eating disorder a name, Ed, so that we can separate it from the individual. When Ed is attempting to infiltrate an individual's healthy self, it is often helpful to the individual and their family to see it as a separate entity from the person's true self. I guide the family and the person struggling that they can be angry, very angry, at Ed. Ed is not their loved one but a wily competitor trying to take over the person. He will say and do anything to protect himself. These statements and actions are symptoms. They aren't lies.

However, it is very difficult for the individual and the family to see that Ed is a separate entity inside the person trying to reach his goal of completely taking over the individual's healthy self. Ed was there when Jon hid weights to inflate his weigh-ins, when he threw away Pop-Tarts and said he had eaten them, and when he snuck out for runs at 2 a.m. so his parents wouldn't know he was doing this. Helping the family see that this wasn't Jon, but the beast, Ed, allows them to be appropriately angry with Ed and set limits to protect Jon. It helps the family see that they aren't fighting with Jon when he erupts, but they are fighting the beast that is trying to brainwash him. Most importantly, it helps Jon see that his parents love him but just despise Ed.

Separating Ed from the healthy part of Jon was vital for his parents to fight against their opponent. They could see that they were angering and disappointing Ed but that they were doing the healthy thing for their son. They were able to stick to their contracts with their treatment teams and this saved Jon's life.

ED THRIVES IN ISOLATION

So many feelings and thoughts welled up inside of me when I talked with both Jon and Lynn. Their struggle affected me both personally and as a psychologist who treats eating disorders. Jon's story is gut-wrenching and, tragically, typical of those struggling with eating disorders, whether male or female. Because of the open way in which Jon has gone about telling his story, his experience has been, and will continue to be helpful to those struggling with this illness. Much of what Jon and his family faced mirrors what those I have treated confronted. The confusion and isolation that Jon and his family felt during his struggle with the eating disorder is very common, especially for males. There is a stigma in our culture to having a mental illness. There is an additional stigma for males with an eating disorder because it is seen traditionally as a "female problem". Most of the boys and men with this illness do not share their struggle with anyone because they feel ashamed. This shame and consequent isolation make it difficult for the individual and family to get the support they need while battling Ed.

Jenni Schaefer describes just how difficult it is for others to understand the behavior of a person who is struggling with Ed in her book, *Life Without Ed* (2004/2014). On page xxx of her book, she states "From the outside looking in, you can't understand it. From the inside looking out, you can't explain it." I thought of this quote as I read the part in Jon's story about his strained relationship with his roommates while in the throes of the eating disorder. People who haven't had to face Ed don't know what to do when it infiltrates their friend or family member. They might try a few conversations with the individual but usually end up distancing themselves from the struggling person. They can't understand why the person is doing what they're doing. They feel helpless against Ed.

When Jon and his girlfriend broke up and again when he went to school in St. Louis and wasn't doing much socially, Ed was able to take up all of the space in Jon's head. Ed wants you alone so he is the only one talking to you. It makes it so much easier for Ed to win when his is the only voice you hear.

There was such an important turning point in Jon's recovery, not only for Jon, but for his mother, when they weren't isolated with the eating disorder's shame and secrecy. For Jon, it started when he joined a fraternity in college. When other things in life, such as social contacts, start fueling a person, Ed becomes less prominent and, hence, less powerful. It was important for Jon to find a social support system that gave him something in life other than counting calories and miles. As Jon reached out to friends, he recovered.

As Lynn confided in friends and allowed herself to be vulnerable about the battle she was fighting, her shame decreased and her friends sustained her in the long war against Ed. Ed thrives on shame and secrecy. Bringing Ed out into the open is its demise. The more the individual and the family struggling with Ed can voice their struggle, the more Ed will lose.

IF A MARATHON IS GOOD, AN IRON MAN IS BETTER

Jon was the victim of our culture's acceptance of over-exercise as normal. Those around him didn't realize at first that what he was doing was part of an eating disorder. Because our culture is obsessed with training for events, it was easy for Jon's symptoms to be masked as healthy. It is even common for physicians to mistake the low heart rate associated with an eating disorder as a "healthy runner's heart." In one case I treated, the physician told the adolescent and her family that she was not healthy enough to participate in track at school. In fact, the physician said that it was highly dangerous due to the low heart rate associated with her eating disorder. Her parents became upset and threatened the school with a lawsuit if she wasn't allowed to run with her team. This may seem like an extreme example, but it is common for families to misunderstand the danger of over-exercise in our training-obsessed culture.

It wasn't until it was too late that anyone recognized Jon's exercise as a symptom. Jon's family probably saved his life when they gave him the ultimatum to receive treatment or lose financial support. Even though his first attempt at treatment was not successful, the seeds were planted to start fighting the eating disorder thoughts.

WHEN ED WINS

One of the saddest experiences I have had in my professional career was when I was treating an adolescent and her family struggling with anorexia many years ago. The family wasn't ready to hear that their daughter needed hospitalization. I was the first psychologist from whom they had sought treatment. Because they rejected hospitalization, we developed a treatment contract to see if their daughter could comply with gaining from a half to one pound per week for four weeks. She was unable to do this. The family would not seek a higher level of care and I was placed in the unfortunate position of having to discontinue treatment with them as I knew that the outpatient work I was doing was not adequate to fight Ed. They sought multiple treatment professionals after me, who all told the family that she required hospitalization. Eventually they had her hospitalized very late into her illness after Ed's grip was too firmly wrapped around her. She died fifteen years later due to complications from her extended war against Ed.

Her mother and father blamed themselves for not having her hospitalized when it was recommended. When they contacted me after her death and voiced their guilt, I was adamant with them that they could not blame themselves. They just couldn't see the severity of Ed at the time. If they had known what they were up against they would have made a different decision. Ed is a master of trickery. Jon was lucky that his parents could not be fooled. Ed takes too many wonderful individuals and leaves families feeling devastated in his wake of destruction.

I CAN DO IT ON MY OWN

In addition to our culture accepting over-exercise as normal, there is also a movement against taking medication. I explain to individuals and their families struggling with Ed that the eating disorder is two-pronged. The first prong is the behaviors that we witness, such as not eating, losing weight, throwing food away, over-exercising, and purging. The second prong is thought infiltration. These are the silver-tongued messages that Ed tells the person who will ultimately develop the eating disorder. Nobody can see these symptoms and they precede the behavior part of the illness for a long time. Families don't realize that by the time they can witness the behavioral parts of Ed, he has been living inside their loved-one's mind for a long time. His messages start quietly and then become loud. They might start with, "hey, you could lose a little weight and be healthier." Ultimately, they progress to statements like, "if eating few calories is good, eating no calories is better." Or, "if running three miles a day is good, running ten miles is better." The messages continue to escalate in frequency and severity.

We use a scale called total conscious time (TCT) to gauge how much time the individual is engaged in eating disorder thoughts and behaviors. When Jon's sister, Bailey, said she missed his personality, I would have guessed that his total conscious time was about 90%. That means that 90% of his waking hours were spent thinking about or engaging in eating disorder symptoms. So, Bailey was only getting 10% of the old, healthy Jon that she loved. The rest of all of Jon's waking time was spent counting calories and miles. When I ask individuals at various times in their treatment to rank their TCT, I often hear, "it's at 110% because I even dream about it!"

The research shows that the thought part of the eating disorder can be aided with the help of some psychotropic medications such as antidepressants. Individuals who try the medication often say that the medication seems to decrease the volume and power of Ed's voice and they feel that they finally have a fighting chance over Ed. The medication is just one tool in the tool kit that may help the individual fight Ed's voice. Unfortunately, our culture, which can be so entrenched against taking medication, makes it difficult for individuals and families to support the recommendation from medical providers to take medication. The individual struggling with Ed doesn't think they have a problem, and their families often believe that the medication will bring more problems than it will help. After many years of working with individuals struggling with Ed, my opinion is that the benefits of the medication far outweigh any possible side effects. In fact, I believe it is nearly impossible to overcome Ed without the aid of medication.

WHEN ED INFILTRATES YOUR NEIGHBORHOOD

I didn't know Lynn well when she reached out to me about Jon's struggle. She contacted me as a neighbor whom she had heard treats eating disorders. I only knew of her as a very philanthropic member of our community who was always involved in some fundraising activity for underprivileged youth. She phoned me, introduced herself, and told me about Jon's struggle. It had been going on for quite a while and she shared that his lab work showed elevated liver enzymes and bradycardia. Often, but not always, when lab work shows elevated liver enzymes, Ed is already close to winning the war. She also shared that he had discontinued seeing his treatment team who were recommending that he re-engage in treatment. He had not signed releases of information, so his parents couldn't talk to his treatment team. I was absolutely terrified! I understood the gravity of the situation. I know that 15% of those struggling with anorexia will succumb fatally to the illness. I have experienced it twice in my practice, and each time, it was absolutely devastating to the families of the deceased and to me personally and professionally.

When I heard that my neighbor's son was alone with ED at college, four hours away, I knew that Ed was calling all the shots. I didn't know Lynn. I couldn't gauge how much of my panic I should let her see. I knew that it took a lot for Lynn to confide in me. I was afraid that if I came on too strong, I would look like a fanatic trying to kill a fly with a baseball bat. I was afraid that if she saw me this way, she would disregard what I had to say. I was afraid that if I wasn't forthright about the gravity of her situation, Jon could be dead in weeks, if not days. I took a leap of faith, a giant one, and told her I was afraid that Jon would die if they didn't get him into an inpatient facility as soon as possible. I told her that if I were her, I wouldn't wait for the next break in school, but I would call the inpatient facilities immediately and have him hospitalized as soon as possible. I hated to scare her. However, I felt that if I could break her out of her denial, it might save Jon's life. Even as I write this, the tears well up. It is hard as a professional and as a person to watch this illness ravage the lives of my clients, my friends, and their children.

ED TAKES PROFESSIONALS

There have been two times in my career that I have had to reduce my caseload due to the emotional drain that the eating disorder caused. It is extremely difficult to bear witness on a daily basis to people in a fight for their life. One of the hardest parts for me is when the individual and the family believe they are fighting me instead of Ed. Ed tells the individual, "you don't have a problem, that psychologist is crazy!" The family doesn't want to think their child has a problem either. So, it's easier to believe their child and to think that the psychologist and team aren't warranted nor helping. At times the individual and family will combat their psychologist in a very angry way. Although I try not to take it personally, it can be overwhelming. In order to remain in the field, I had to reduce my caseload to eleven clients on two different occasions.

Currently, I no longer treat adolescents. After battling Ed with adolescents and their families for twenty years, I realized that Ed had defeated my ability to fight for that age group. It was too hard to confront the adolescent and the entire family system anymore. So, for the past eight years I have treated solely those over the age of eighteen who struggle with Ed and have supervised therapists who are treating adolescents and their families. It is so much easier to fight Ed in adolescents as a supervisor than to be on the front lines. Ed is a formidable opponent who often creates burnout in many professionals. It is very common for those who treat Ed to cease seeing those struggling with Ed at a certain point in their career. They welcome people struggling with depression, anxiety, and trauma, anything other than an eating disorder. Ed takes causalities of all types.

AM I FIGHTING MY CHILD OR ED?

The strength of the Sestak family to insist that Jon receive a higher level of care in the face of Ed is admirable! I'm sure they felt like they were fighting their son. Because Jon didn't want to be hospitalized, they had to separate healthy Jon from Ed in order to enforce hospitalization. When reading both Lynn and Jon's accounts about the events that led to his hospitalization, I had to put their book down and cry. I cried when reading about Jon's hospital roommate who later succumbed to Ed. I cried for Jon, a 20-year-old man, so young, who had to see a friend die from the very disease he was battling. I cried for the two clients I once treated who would later lose their battles to Ed.

I will never forget the day in 1990 when one of my supervisors told me, "If you treat eating disorders, you will have clients who die. Are you ready for this?" As a naïve 26-year-old one year from getting my PhD I said, "Sure." Over the years, much of the professional supervision I have received has been about dealing with these losses. Now, when I supervise therapists starting in my field today, I find myself on the other side of that conversation.

THERE ARE NO PERFECT PEOPLE. THERE ARE NO PERFECT PARENTS.

Jon was at a particularly hard age for parents to join the fight against Ed. When the individual struggling with the eating disorder is over eighteen, he can check himself in or out of treatment and refuse to authorize the release information to anyone other than himself. When I have worked with families whose child is a minor, I implore them to get the hospitalizations or higher levels of care needed prior to their child turning eighteen. After that, as with Jon's parents, money is usually the only point of leverage to enforce limits against Ed. Not paying for Jon's ticket home from the hospital when he discharged himself was probably counterintuitive to his parents. However, it was one of the steps that helped Jon recover from Ed. The Sestaks persevered but I'm sure it took a toll on them. Loving him and hugging him when he came home but withholding financial support had to be excruciating! Tough love is hard. Setting financial limits with love and without anger is difficult. Every family should know that nobody does this perfectly. Every parent will lose it and yell at times. It is understandable when fighting an opponent like Ed and when the consequence is their child's life.

I truly believe that Jon's family saved his life when they took my advice to have him admitted into a higher level of care. At that time, we didn't have any options for a higher level of care in Kansas City. I can't imagine how overwhelming it must have been for Jon's family, and every other family in Kansas City, to hear that the closest treatment facilities were four to ten hours away in St. Louis, Denver, or Chicago. When I have recommended to clients' families over the years that they take their child to one of these cities and leave them there, they looked at me like I was crazy! They couldn't imagine sending their child away from home when their child was so ill.

I can't even imagine how terrifying it was to leave Jon in Denver and the strength that it must have taken the Sestak family to entrust their beloved son to people they don't know, then board a plane and fly hundreds of miles away from him to return home. I can only imagine how much faith and courage it took for them and for all of the other families who have had to do this. I also understand the relief that must be a part of that experience because the families hope that they will be on the road to seeing their healthy child back again.

NOBODY GAVE US A HANDBOOK ON HOW TO FIGHT ED

Lynn and Steve did a fantastic job in honoring Jon as an adult and danced a fine line by supporting Jon's healthy decisions but refusing to support Ed. Although we recommend that all families have a separate family therapist to guide them in the fight against Ed, many families refuse to see one due to the enormous amount of time and money that is already going into the individual's treatment. However, when families do enlist their own family therapist it greatly enhances the treatment outcome! Kudos to Lynn and Steve for reaching out and getting guidance from an objective therapist.

ED BEGINS TO LOSE

I had a huge smile when I read that Jon almost stole bran crackers. Thank goodness Ed encouraged Jon to do this. I think this was the point where Ed began to lose his war with Jon. Ed encourages people to steal such items as food, diet pills, diuretics or laxatives to fuel their eating disorder. Because this behavior was so foreign to Jon's moral compass, he recognized that Ed had crossed the line. He did something so outrageous that Jon could not reconcile his actions with the way he saw himself. This was a turning point for Jon, the beginning of his own internal desire to overcome Ed. It is important to note that if Jon's parents had not set the financial limits they had, Jon would never have experienced this internal struggle.

There is no "right "way to recover. Everyone's journey is different. If the person struggling with Ed is underweight, part of recovery will be regaining and maintaining a healthy weight. It is important to note that having a dietitian who specializes in eating disorders guide the refeeding process is crucial. This is because the individual is in one of their most physically fragile times during the recovery process when they are re-gaining weight. If weight is regained in an unhealthy way, refeeding syndrome can develop, a complication of which can lead to death. It was important for Jon's parents to have Jon see a dietician during his recovery process.

My hat goes off to the dietitians who treat eating disorders! If a psychologist feels under attack from a client or client's family, it is the dieticians who bear the brunt of Ed's wrath. They are the unlucky individuals on the treatment team who directly contradict Ed's dietary messages. When the individual says, "I can eat six extra crackers," it is the dietician who says, "No, you must eat twelve." It is the dietician who tells the parents they must ensure that their child consumes the daily recommended amount of food. This creates tension and causes the family to debate about whether the dietician is doing a good job. It is very common for a family to see more than one dietician during the course of treatment because they have to hear the same messages from different providers to understand that they are getting accurate medical advice. It is a relief when the individual is in the later stages of recovery and they start to see the dietician as an ally rather than an enemy.

As Jon fueled his body with food, his brain was able to think better and more adequately combat Ed. When our brains are starved, we are not thinking clearly. Ed has such an advantage when we are not fueling our bodies appropriately.

AM I REALLY RECOVERED?

When I first read Jon and Lynn's book, I found myself up until 2 a.m., wrought with emotion. I found myself crying so hard at times, I had to put the book down to let it out. The next day I called Lynn and Jon to meet with them to give them my impressions. Jon asked during this meeting, "am I recovered? I mean, am I truly recovered enough to write this book from the perspective of a healthy person?" There are divergent opinions about whether full recovery is possible and what it looks like. Personally, I believe in full recovery as I see it every day in my practice! I told Jon he may not be exactly where he wants to be, the Jon before Ed, but he is much closer than when Ed had almost total control over him.

I told Jon that he will keep getting better and better over time. It takes a long time to remove all of the little tendrils that Ed had created in his brain. I am confident that he will find less and less rigidity with food over time. I told him there will be a day when he will be able to eat two-for-one burgers at Johnny's with his dad without any second thoughts. I am confident in telling Jon this because I see it happening all of the time! I told Jon, and I truly believe this, that he will be fully recovered. He will be the healthy self that he was with his full, wonderful personality back. And, one last thing that I would tell Jon is that he will actually be stronger because of Ed. I know that this may sound crazy, but individuals who have recovered from an eating disorder are more insightful, wise, and empathetic than they were prior to their illness. It is the one gift that Ed leaves behind.

Jon mentioned that he feels guilty for all of the pain he put his family through. Those who develop eating disorders are usually individuals who hate to be a burden to others. They are typically perfectionistic, goal-oriented, people pleasers who will die with their boots on trying to do the right thing to take care of everyone else. It is very normal for them to feel guilty about the pain, money, and energy that their families put into their treatment. It is usually an ongoing struggle for the individual in treatment to let their family know how much help they need. I have seen families do what Jon's family did, anything they could to help fight the illness, no matter the expense or sacrifices they have to make.

I am asked Jon's question, "am I recovered enough?", when clients want to speak about their recovery. They often feel they are not recovered enough to publicly tell their story. I confront this fallacy head on. I believe that not sharing their story contributes to the shame and silence around the struggle with Ed. It is one of Ed's last attempts to keep the person quiet and isolated with only his voice speaking to them. I don't mean that I think that everybody who has had an eating disorder needs to be an advocate for the disease, but if the person desires to speak out, and Ed is trying to talk him out of it, then Ed needs to be silenced.

Faith is often an important component in recovery, just like it was for Lynn and Jon. Many families feel great support by leaning on their faith and on others who worship with them. Lynn was able to be vulnerable and expose her biggest struggle, Jon's eating disorder, with her Bible study group. This supportive group helped her persevere in the war against Ed.

THE WAR AGAINST ED IN THE PRESS

It is always difficult for me, as a friend and neighbor, to know how much to ask after a person calls me for help in seeking treatment for themselves or a family member. I know that most of them feel very exposed and vulnerable and often don't want to talk about this with me again once I help them locate a psychologist. After Lynn reached out to me, it appeared to me that she did not want many questions about where they were with Jon and his battle. I could be very wrong about that, but I didn't ask questions. So, I really knew nothing about where Jon was with his struggle when I received a telephone call from a reporter with our local newspaper, the <u>Kansas City Star</u>. He told me that Jon had inquired about writing a story regarding his struggle with his eating disorder and that his mother and Jon had been interviewed for the paper. He told me that they had given him my name as someone he might want to interview. I received permission from both Jon and his mother to speak to the reporter.

I admired Jon and Lynn so much for their desire to make their story public! Jon had such bravery and courage to open up about his struggle, especially as a male who had an eating disorder.

Because Jon is a gifted, smart, well-liked, athletic, masculine man, I think it hit every reader that this can happen to anyone. After his story came out, I couldn't believe the response that the Sestaks and I received from the story. Many called to say that they felt their son or husband was struggling with the same disorder. I wasn't surprised when the <u>Kansas City Star</u> followed up on the story a year or so later. The reporter told me they did the follow up because it was the most talked about story in the history of the <u>Kansas City Star</u>. Jon's story has helped others reach out for the treatment they need. I admire Jon and his entire family for their willingness to continue to fight Ed even after it is no longer a daily struggle. Their fight against Ed and their willingness to publicize it has changed the landscape in Kansas City for males struggling with eating disorders. I am truly honored to have been a very small part of their story. They are heroes who are strongly admired by me and those in my field.

BAILEY'S PERSPECTIVE

I am Bailey, Jon's little sister. Before I share my experience with my big brother's battle with anorexia, I will share a little bit about me. Throughout school, I was a straight-A (with the occasional, dreaded A-) student, perfectionist, and major people-pleaser. I enjoyed listening more than talking and was careful not to hurt anybody's feelings. I was actively involved in several student organizations, competitively danced, and landed a spot on the gymnastics team. Based on the statistics, I was the one who was supposed to succumb to anorexia, not Jon. I constantly found myself asking questions like "Why Jon?" "Why not me?" "How can I fix this?" I never found the answer to any of these questions.

I had always looked up to Jon, and still do. After all, he was my "cooler" older brother who made all the right moves. He was athletic and well-known by all. He was humorous, friendly, and the life-of-the-party. I felt special when Jon would let me hang out with his friends for five minutes. He was and still is one of my best friends. When the anorexia hit, though, the old Jon disappeared.

I was going into my senior year of high school when Jon's disease first sprouted. As a high schooler, I always imagined senior year to be "the best year yet!" Although it was an enjoyable year, my brother's disease and the negative effects it was having on my family was always present in the back of my mind. Whenever I hung out with friends, I found myself feeling guilty about not being home. I felt guilty for not doing more, even though there was not more for me to do. The weight of this "secret" really took its toll, and I found myself crying in my room a lot.

Simply put, Jon stopped being Jon. When I came home from a friend's house late at night, I would peek in the basement window to find Jon researching healthy recipes on his computer. One 105-degree summer day, I was lying out with a few girlfriends when I saw Jon running (sprinting) around the four-mile lake. At meals, I watched him cut meat into dime-sized pieces before finally eating one piece. We all watched in amazement at his eating habits. Family time became all about Jon and eating. We had family interventions that did not seem to spark any change in Jon. After a while, I stopped asking "where's Jon?" because I knew exactly where he was, working out. Things were hard.

No one tells you about the emotions you experience when a loved one develops an eating disorder. I was frustrated. I was angry. I was sad. I was concerned. I was disappointed when my parents' interventions were not working. At one point, I began mourning the loss of my brother because death seemed too close.

As anorexia nervosa continued to take over my brother, I headed off to college. I felt guilty about leaving my family when they needed me the most. Coming home for breaks and holidays was difficult. I think the phrase, "If I don't see it, it didn't happen" is applicable here. I never understood the severity and extent of this eating disorder on my brother until I saw him. Many times, I just wanted to stuff a doughnut down his throat. I couldn't understand why he couldn't just eat, especially when most Americans have the opposite problem.

I am proud of my parents. They handled Jon's situation extremely well and always wanted to do what was best for everyone. They dealt with stereotyped judgement and misunderstanding from many. They never made me feel like it was "my problem." As Jon went to Saint Louis University, they worked hard to separate my life from Jon's, which I think Jon appreciated.

I wish I had more advice to share. As Jon mentioned, you cannot make someone change if they are unwilling to change. I did my best to be a support and friend to my brother. Even though life was changing and family talks with him seemed to go nowhere, I worked hard to maintain my relationship with him. Let me tell you, it's hard watching someone you love so much turn into an irrational stranger.

I was scared of losing my brother. Solutions seemed to be scarce. There was nothing I could do. I did what I could do to be the best sister to my brother. He felt a lot of tension and concern from others, so I avoided talking about ED at all costs. I just wanted him to be happy AND alive.

Fortunately, God did the rest. He put the right therapists, the right treatment centers, and the right events in Jon's life to ultimately heal him from the burden of ED. I am thankful for God's ability to heal and bring my brother back. Male anorexia ultimately strengthened my family's relationship with one another, and I hope the same happens for you and your family. Pray and remain positive. Everything happens for a reason.

STEVE'S PERSPECTIVE

I would never proclaim to be the perfect husband or father. Actually, far from it. But, when it comes to the safety and security of my family, I would do just about anything. During my youth, I excelled at sports and was generally a very good student. I never got into big trouble, at least nothing anybody can prove. I played football in college, but would define myself as one of those who went professional in something other than my sport. I spent my entire thirty-year career in the Business Consulting industry; first as a partner at a major international firm, then as the founder and chief executive of my own business. Solving complex problems is not something new to me. It is what I have done my entire career. But, when it came to solving the irrational eating disorder that inflicted my son, I was at a total loss.

Despite my busy work schedule, I coached Jon's soccer teams for several years until his talents exceeded my coaching abilities. As he progressed through various club teams, I often spent weekends at his regional soccer tournaments and loved the time we spent together in the hotel rooms and seeking out the unique food experiences that the cities we visited had to offer. After his team won one of their state championship games, while the other players were celebrating together on the field, my son jumped the fence, ran up to where I was sitting, and gave me a big hug. That moment will always stick in my mind as the point where I knew that all of the time we had spent together honing his skills had made a difference and was appreciated by him. When it came to track, I had to defer to my wife. She was a track star in high school and had a better appreciation of this sort of individual sport. The notion of achieving your "personal best" meant little to me as I excelled at team sports where achievement is measured in wins and losses. Regardless, I enjoyed watching Jon excel in that sport, as well.

Anyone who plays sports knows that there is always someone out there who is faster, stronger, or simply better than you are. They also know that there will be a time when your days of competitive sports come to an end. Some get to choose that time while, for others, that time is chosen for them. I stopped playing college football my junior year because I had lost respect for the coaches I was playing for. But, I still wonder whether I had made the right decision. After a successful high school career, I was excited that Jon had been sought out by several colleges to play soccer and had set a new goal of competing in triathlons. He was always a great runner, but taught himself to be a better swimmer and biker. When it came to sports, his work ethic was impressive and definitely exceeded those of his father.

It was during his preparation for his first triathlon that I noticed there was a problem. I recognized his frustration with "hitting the wall" during his senior year of track, but was glad to see him put that behind him and focus on a new challenge. I have never personally aspired to complete a triathlon, so I attributed his restrictive eating and weight loss to the excessive training. I believed that things would return to normal once that event was completed. Never would I imagine that the seeds of anorexia had already been planted, and we would be in for the most challenging period of our parental responsibilities. I had little doubt that we would once again be able to share in our regular burger nights at Johnny's Tavern or take advantage of all of the great barbeque restaurants that Kansas City has to offer. Once again, when I played competitive sports and was told to gain weight, the solution was simple… "just eat more!"

I remember telling Jon goodbye as he headed off to college with my wife and daughter. I was excited for him as he embarked on this next journey, but could not help but feel a little scared as it had become clear that he needed some professional help with his eating disorder. I was optimistic that, with this help and the multitude of eating options that college life provides, he would quickly regain his weight. But, when I first visited and took him shopping at the local Sam's Club, it became evident that the problem had become much bigger. He did not want the typical "college junk food" and preferred large quantities of pickles, refried beans, and oatmeal. What's wrong with an occasional Pop-Tart, Twinkie, or some ice cream? Despite my coaxing, he would politely decline. At least I am glad to know now that I did not spend money on those things only to have him throw them out.

What ensued over the next year is beyond anything I could have expected. Visits to college always left me wondering what had happened to the son I loved. Time spent at home was often disrupted by family interventions, new contracts, and emotional outbursts. I was shocked to see what he would voluntarily put on his plate and the things he would do to avoid spending time with his family and friends. While we often spent our time together throwing the football in the park across the street, many of these conversations anchored on negotiations regarding his excessive exercise and odd eating behaviors. When we were finally able to convince him to get the professional help he desperately needed, he did not take is seriously and often checked himself out against our pleas to continue. This was not the son with the work ethic I was so proud of.

As I mentioned before, I would do just about anything for my family. It was not until we attended a family day at the treatment center in Denver that I realized that he could actually die from this disease. After coming to grips with that reality, I was prepared to do whatever it took to cure my son of his eating disorder. However, what I know now is that, similar to other addictions, the cure can only begin when the person inflicted decides to change behaviors. I personally do not care what triggered Jon to cure himself of this disease; I am just glad it happened and have been amazed at his recovery over the past several years. I am glad to have my old son back. While I was always proud of Jon's accomplishments in sports, academics, and other endeavors, I am even more proud of his tenacity in curing himself of his eating disorder. I am also proud of his willingness to share his story and help others who are inflicted with this disease. As a father, your primary job is to protect your family. While I desperately wanted to protect Jon when he was inflicted with this disease, I now know that the most I could do was provide love and support. Now that he is better, we often share a laugh over some of the things we tried. Jon commented that he had noticed that I had lost some hair during this ordeal. I am not sure whether any of my hair has grown back as he had indicated, but I thank him for salvaging the last few I have left. I guess every child challenges their parents in ways they could never imagine, but never would I have imagined dealing with the challenges of an eating disorder.

Looking back at this episode, I owe my wife a tremendous debt of gratitude for her diligence in researching this disease and seeking out the best treatment for our son. But, most of all, for her compassionate, yet stern approach to confronting manifestations of the disease while providing love and support for our son. Her faith in God was instrumental during this process. She claims that her active involvement with our children's activities might have been a trigger. But, I would have to disagree and am grateful for the engaged role she played in the raising of our children. While this disease can put a strain on any marriage, I believe we have emerged from it with more love and respect for each other. I thank God for her and for his grace in not allowing our son to be another fatality of this illogical disease.

To a father of a child inflicted with this disease, my advice might sound irrational. But, then again, so is an eating disorder to any normal person. Encourage your children to excel at sports, academics, or whatever interests they have. Celebrate wins and other achievements, but keep them in perspective. Capitalize on losses or setbacks as they are part of ordinary life. Recognize the transitions of adolescents and the pressures that society places on perfection. Talk openly about the problems they are facing while offering advice and not judging their feelings. As men, we are expected to protect our children and always know the answer or how to solve the problem. When we don't, we often resort to the primeval instinct of rage, threats and punishments. That might work when confronting a rational situation. But, once again, an eating disorder is not a rational disease. It takes patience, persistence, and consistency to overcome. Like many of you, I feel fortunate to have smart, athletic, and social children who have high aspirations for what they want to accomplish in life. Unfortunately, this disease lurks in those same types of children and preys off the pressures they feel to achieve those accomplishments.

SUPPORTIVE BIBLE VERSES

Life Application Study Bible

Ephesians 6:10 A final word: Be strong with the Lord's might power.

Ephesians 4:31-32 Get rid of all bitterness, rage, anger, harsh words, and slander, as well as all types of malicious behavior. Instead, be kind to each other, tenderhearted, forgiving one another, just as God through Christ has forgiven you.

Luke 12-29-31 And don't worry about food—what to eat and drink. Don't worry whether God will provide it for you. These things dominate the thoughts of most people, but your Father already knows your needs. He will give you all you need from day to day if you make the Kingdom of God your primary concern.

James 1:5-6 If you need wisdom—if you want to know what God wants you to do—ask him, and he will gladly tell you. He will not resent your asking. But when you ask him, be sure that you really expect him to answer, for a doubtful mind is as unsettled as a wave of the sea that is driven and tossed by the wind.

Nahum 1:7 The Lord is good. When trouble comes, he is a strong refuge. And he knows everyone who trusts in him.

Matthew 6:34 So don't worry about tomorrow, for tomorrow will bring its own worries. Today's trouble is enough for today.

Proverbs 19:21 You can make plans, but the Lord's purpose will prevail.

Isaiah 55:8-9 My thoughts are completely different from yours, says the Lord. And my ways are far beyond anything you could imagine. For just as the heavens are higher than the earth, so are my ways higher than your ways and my thoughts higher than your thoughts.

Exodus 14:14 The Lord himself will fight for you. You won't have to lift a finger in your defense!

Romans 8:26 And the Holy Spirit helps us in our distress. For we don't even know what we should pray for, nor how we should pray. But the Holy Spirit prays for us with groanings that cannot be expressed in words.

1Peter 4:12-13 Dear friends, don't be surprised at the fiery trials you are going through, as if something strange were happening to you. Instead, be very glad—because these trials will make you partners with Christ in his suffering, and afterward you will have the wonderful joy of sharing his glory when it is displayed to all the world.

Proverbs 3:5-6 Trust in the Lord with all your heart; do not depend on your own understanding. Seek his will in all you do, and he will direct your paths.

Psalm 30:2 O Lord my God, I cried to you for help and you restored my health.

1Corininthians 6:19-20 Or don't you know that your body is the temple of the Holy Spirit, who lives in you and was given to you by God? You do not belong to yourself. For God bought you with a high price. So you must honor God with your body.

Philippians 4:6-7 Don't worry about anything; instead pray about everything. Tell God what you need, and thank him for all he has done. If you do this, you will experience God's peace, which is far more wonderful than the human mind can understand. His peace will guard your hearts and minds as you live in Christ Jesus.

Philippians 4:13 For I can do everything with the help of Christ who gives me the strength I need.

Isaiah 40:29 He gives power to those who are tired and worn out; he offers strength to the weak.

Psalm 34:18 The Lord is close to the brokenhearted; he rescues those who are crushed in spirit.

Psalm 34:4 I prayed to the Lord, and he answered me, freeing me from all my fears.

REFERENCES

Allen, K.L., Byrne, S.M., Oddy, W.H., & Crosby, R.D. (2013). DSM-IV-TR and DSM5 eating disorders in adolescents: Prevalence, stability, and psychosocial correlates in a population-based sample of male and female adolescents. *Journal of Abnormal Psychology, 122* (3), 720-732.

Bachner-Melman, R., Zohar, A.H., Ebstein, R.P., Elizur, Y., & Constantini, N. (2006). How anorexic-like are the symptom and personality profiles of aesthetic athletes? *Medicine & Science in Sports & Exercise, 38* (4), 628-636.

Brotsky, S.R. (2014). Understanding stages of change in the recovery process. *Eating Disorders Recovery Today, Fall 2009, 7* (4), ©2009 Gürze Books. Retrieved July 27, 2016 from Eating Disorders Recovery Today. http://www.eatingdisordersrecoverytoday.com/understanding-stages-of-change-in-the-recovery-process/

Cohn, L. (2013). "Male Gender Roles and Other Sociocultural Factors in Navigating Access to Treatment," International Conference on Eating Disorders (plenary session), Montreal, Canada.

Eisenberg, D., Nicklett, E.J., Roeder, K., & Kirz, N.E. (2011). Eating disorders symptoms among college students: prevalence, persistence, correlates, and treatment-seeking. *Journal of American College Health, 59* (8), 700-707.

Fussell, J. (2013, August 23). Their secret pain. *The Kansas City Star*.

Feldman, M. B., & Meyer, I.H. (2007). Eating disorders in diverse, lesbian, gay, and bisexual populations. *International Journal of Eating Disorders, 40* (3), 218-226.

Fichter, M. M., & Quadflieg, N. (2016). Mortality in eating disorders – Results of a large prospective clinical longitudinal study. *International Journal of Eating Disorders*, Epub ahead of print.

Gueguen, J., Godart, N., Chambry, J., Brun-Eberentz, A., Foulon, C., Divac, S.M.,... Huas, C. (2012). Severe anorexia nervosa in men: Comparison with severe AN in women and analysis of mortality. *International Journal of Eating Disorders, 45* (4), 537–545.

Hausenblas, H.A., & Downs, D.S. (2002). Relationship among sex, imagery, and exercise dependence symptoms. *Psychology of Addictive Behavior, 16* (2), 169-172.

Hudson, J.I., Hiripi, E., Pope, H.G., & Kessler, R.C. (2007). The prevalence and correlates of eating disorders in the national comorbidity survey replication. *Biological Psychiatry, 61* (3), 348-358.

Jones, M. (n.d.). Factors that may contribute to eating disorders. National Eating Disorders Association. Retrieved July 25, 2016, from https://www.nationaleatingdisorders.org/factors-may-contribute-eating-disorders

Mond, J.M., Mitchison, D., & Hay, P. (2014) Prevalence and implications of eating disordered behavior in men in Cohn, Lemberg.

National Association of Males with Eating Disorders. (n.d.) Anorexia nervosa. Retrieved July 26, 2016, from http://namedinc.org/?page_id=32

National Eating Disorders Association. (n.d.) Anorexia nervosa in males. Retrieved July 25, 2016, from https://www.nationaleatingdisorders.org/anorexia-nervosa-males

National Eating Disorders Association. (n.d.) Anorexia nervosa warning signs. Retrieved July 25, 2016, from https://www.nationaleatingdisorders.org/anorexia-nervosa

Raevuori, A., Keski-Rahkonen, A., & Hoek, H. W. (2014). A review of eating disorders in males. *Current Opinions on Psychiatry*, *27* (6), 426-430.

Schaefer, Jenni (2014). Introduction. *Life without ed* (pp. xxx). New York: McGraw Hill Education. (Original work published 2004).

Smink, F. E., van Hoeken, D., & Hoek, H. W. (2012). Epidemiology of eating disorders: Incidence, prevalence and mortality rates. *Current Psychiatry Reports, 14*(4), 406-414.

Steinhausen, H.C. (2002). The outcome of anorexia nervosa in the 20th century. *American Journal of Psychiatry*, *159*(8), 1284-1293.

Sundgot-Borgen, J., & Torstveit, M.K. (2004). Prevalence of eating disorders in elite athletes is higher than in the general population. *Clinical Journal of Sport Medicine*, *14* (1), 25-32.

Wade, T.D., Keski-Rahkonen, A., & Hudson, J. (2011). Epidemiology of eating disorders. In M.Tsuang & M. Tohen (Eds.), *Textbook in Psychiatric Epidemiology* (3rd ed.) (pp. 343-360) New York: Wiley.

Weltzin, T.E., (2014a). Males with eating disorders and exercise clinical characteristics and treatment. *Gurze Salucore Eating Disorders Resource Catalogue*, edcatalogue.com

Weltzin, T., Carlson, T., Cornella-Carlson, T., Fitzpatrick, M.E., Kennington, B., Bean, P., & Jefferies, C. (2014b). Treatment issues and outcomes for males with eating disorders. *Eating Disorders 2012, 20* (5), 444-459 in Cohn, Lemberg.

Zucker, N.L., Womble, L.G., Williamson, D.A., & Perrin, L. (1999). Protective factors for eating disorders in female college athletes. *Eating Disorders: The Journal of Treatment and Prevention, 7* (3), 207-218.

BIOGRAPHY
Michelle Micsko, PhD.

Dr. Micsko, Licensed Psychologist in both Kansas and Missouri and specialist in treating Eating Disorders, dedicates her career in Kansas City to the widespread issues of compulsive and disordered eating. Since 1987, Dr. Micsko has provided individual, family, and group psychotherapy for adolescents and adults specializing in the treatment of eating issues and body image concerns. The National Speaking of Women's Health Foundation honored her in 2003 with an award of distinction for her contributions to Eating Disorder treatment in Kansas City. She co-founded InSight Counseling, LLC comprised of highly trained specialists who are passionate in treating those who are struggling with Eating Disorders. She facilitates seminars locally and nationally for teens and adults on topics related to disordered eating and provides training and ongoing supervision to professionals who treat Eating Disorders. Dr. Micsko is an advocate for those struggling with Eating Disorders and has been a spokesperson in this capacity publicly via television, radio and newspaper. She has been instrumental in bringing many nationally known speakers to Kansas City to help further public and professional education regarding eating issues. For over two decades, Dr. Micsko has been the President of the nonprofit Body Balance Coalition, a foundation designed to promote education and awareness regarding eating issues to both professionals and the general public. She is also serving as an ambassador for the Binge Eating Disorder Association, a national foundation focused on providing leadership, recognition, prevention, and treatment of binge eating disorder (BED) and associated weight stigma. Dr. Micsko is also married and the mother of two children.

www.ingramcontent.com/pod-product-compliance
Lightning Source LLC
Chambersburg PA
CBHW050538280326
41933CB00011B/1631